Hypnotic Language

Its Structure And Use

John J. Burton EdD
&
Bobby G. Bodenhamer DMin

Crown House Publishing Limited
www.crownhouse.co.uk
www.crownhousepublishing.com

First published in the UK by

Crown House Publishing Limited
Crown Buildings, Bancyfelin, Carmarthen, Wales, SA33 5ND, UK
www.crownhouse.co.uk

and

Crown House Publishing LLC
6 Trowbridge Drive, Suite 5, Bethel, CT 06801-2858, USA
www.crownhousepublishing.com

British Library Cataloguing-in-Publication Data
A catalogue entry for this book is available
from the British Library.

ISBN 978-184590285-8

LCCN 2009928380

Printed and bound in the USA

Contents

Acknowledgements

I would like to extend my gratitude to the fine people at Crown House Publishing. This includes Martin Roberts, Bridget Shine and Matt Pearce whose patience and skill allowed this book to become a reality.

I would also like to extend my appreciation to Bob Bodenhamer for immeasurable contributions and guidance.

I would also like to thank Michael Hall for sharing his mind, giving feedback and for his written contributions to this work.

I would like also to acknowledge Milton Erickson for his crucial contributions toward making hypnosis what it is today. What a fine model for combining genius with compassion.

Finally, I would like to express my appreciation to the source and foundation who makes all available.

John Burton EdD
2000

Foreword

Imagine meeting someone on the street or in a coffee shop, or at your office tomorrow who whispers something important to you. They take you aside for just a moment and say,

> "You can, by just saying some words, send people into wild and wonderful places and give them altered experiences, and possibly change their lives, empower them with new abilities, and much more."

Would you believe that person? Would such magic and power seem possible? By just talking?

There is a language that makes this possible. We call it the language of trance. Such language invites us out of any present moment and into a state of the mind where we 'go inside' and see, hear, feel, smell, taste and experience an altered reality. Did I say, 'altered'? That's probably over-stating it. 'Different' may be more accurate. We call this state 'hypnosis' yet that too miscommunicates more than it communicates. Because, as Dr Burton will show in this book of language patterns, we cannot not experience trance-states. To 'think' about another time and place is to transition out of this moment and to hallucinate another time, whether past or future.

That language hypnotizes, you know well when you think about it. Any good storyteller, minister, mother, novel, etc. can invite us out of the present and into a world constructed in our mind. From the outside all of this seems mysterious. Even spooky. From the outside the person seems to be asleep (hence the word hypnotism). But from the inside, ah, from the inside—your mind is never more alert and awake, more in control and expansive. And it all occurs upon the wings of language.

But how does language do this? Wherein lies the magic? What kinds of words facilitate this near magic-like process? This book will first of all give you an extensive understanding of some of the mental or cognitive processes that make it so and then will put into your hands some of the most powerful hypnotic language patterns. In this work, John uses his extensive knowledge of

Neuro-Linguistics and Neuro-Semantics—his field of expertise—child developmental psychology, Gestalt psychology and even Meta-states.

Meta-states? You know, a state of mind or emotion that relates to another state as when you begin to feel really curious about learning about hypnotic language patterns. The learning state is one thing, feeling excited and full of anticipation about your learning is a higher state. And now that you can go in and make sense of that, I'm sure that you can just as easily appreciate your skills at feeling excited as you expect to expand your skills in the process of this learning, can you not?

If that doesn't invite you to trance out, we only have to add another level, or seven more. Each shift upwards invites you into a hypnotic state as the referents do not exist 'out there,' but 'in there' (imagine me pointing to your head, ah, another invitation to trance!). See, it's inevitable. Accordingly, Dr Burton along with Dr Bob Bodenhamer have taken Meta-states as the newest NLP model and used it to articulate many new language patterns in the context of assisting people to make the kind of transformations in their mental maps that will give them a new lease on life.

Should you buy this book? *Yes*, of course, if you're interested in how language works its magic. Yes, if you're interested in becoming more playful with your language skills. Yes, if you're interested in inducing powerful states that can enable others to become more empowered and skilled, buy this book. In fact, it seems to me that from psycho-hypnotists, psychotherapists, coaches, consultants, to teachers, writers, trainers, marketers, advertisers, parents, lawyers, politicians, many will want to get their hands on this volume. But that's just a suggestion.

L. Michael Hall PhD
Colorado

Preface

In 1996, I received a call from John Burton who had an interest in taking the Neuro-Linguistic Programming (NLP) training that I offered. I learned that John worked as a Licensed Professional Counselor (LPC) in Greenville, SC. This thrilled me, as I love training counselors in the skills of NLP. Soon John was with me in the NLP summer practitioner training course.

We were not very far along in the training before I realized that in John Burton I had a unique student. John brought with him immense knowledge and keen insight. I learned that John received a doctorate from Vanderbilt, a highly acclaimed university in Nashville, Tennessee. John did his doctoral studies primarily in the field of developmental psychology.

During the NLP master practitioner training, I and the other students stood in awe as John began delivering hypnotic language patterns. I have had other students who could outdo their trainer with hypnotic languaging. But, never, and I mean never, have I heard language patterns flow from a person as they did from John.

John comes up each year and teaches the hypnosis training of my master practitioner training. He was up last December for my present students. Three months have passed since John last taught and those students are still talking about John Burton and their amazement at his skill.

Thanks to Crown House Publishing, you now have access to his genius. I know that on the front of this book you have both our names as the author. However, I cannot lay claim to the genius of this book. Inside these covers you will find numerous examples of 'doing hypnosis'. Most of the patterns come from actual client sessions.

Also, in the first three chapters you will learn the 'how' of hypnosis. Indeed, you are in for a real treat and for an understanding of 'how' hypnosis works based on the latest in the cognitive sciences and from developmental psychology.

Indeed, I am honored to have been just a small part of this work.

Bobby G. Bodenhamer DMin

Part One

The Three Facets
that Allow the Mind to be
Susceptible to Hypnotic Language Patterns

Introduction

Hypnosis and the Cognitive Pathways it Travels

Suppose you treat a mistake, any mistake, like an oil spill at sea? What then? The oil recovery team will place barriers around the oil to contain the spill. As you imagine this, notice how the ocean outside the containers remains clear and clean. Also, knowing that oil is lighter than water and floats, resting only on the surface. This allows the water underneath the oil to remain clear and clean.

This means that the only task remaining is to remove the oil by skimming the oil from the sea… so that you can see it disappear slowly or quickly and as you do, noticing the feeling as the oil departs to leave more and more sea to see and feel…the clear and clean return. Now, how will you enjoy the sea sight as you set your sights on your future?

I used the above hypnotic language pattern with a client who came in complaining of depression. He had a foolproof way of creating depression. Any time he made a mistake he would generalize from the mistake and contaminate his whole self. He would conclude, 'I made a mistake, therefore I am a bad person'.

Does that sound familiar? He was an expert in making a bad person out of himself. He would stew for days in self-criticism, which resulted in constant feelings of depression. A vicious circle of self-criticism, pessimism and self-depreciation would put him in and keep him in a state of depression. He had the depression strategy down pat. Once he heard this pattern, it changed his way of viewing his mistakes.

From this point on, he saw any mistakes he made as isolated errors and relied on his positive memories of his many successes to nullify these mistakes. Instead of generalizing from his mistake to the whole of himself, he generalized to the part making the error and thereby brought his successful self to bear on this part. In doing this, he thus nullified any depression (a Meta-stating process—more about Meta-states later).

He reported in our next session how he had made some errors, but was not upset by them, rather he went right on working toward solutions. He stated that, for a change, he was enjoying being in a good mood and that he was feeling very competent. That was our last session.

A follow-up over six months later revealed that he continued feeling good and no longer had any of those self-criticism spells. He even began resuming some of his favorite hobbies that he'd given up while trying so hard to prove his competence.

What happens in the mind that empowers it in such a way that it can hear a few hypnotic words, and the listener turns her world totally around? You will find out as you learn the concepts in these first three introductory chapters.

All communication invites the receiver into a hypnotic trance.

In this text, a hypnotic state or trance refers to a focusing of attention on a thought, idea, concept, thing, etc. which excludes all other focusing on anything else.

It is important to recognize that all communication invites the receiver into a hypnotic trance. Whenever we make a statement, the person hearing our statement cannot help but respond to those words and to the thoughts that they stimulate. They will connect some meaning to what we say, and, at least for a moment, as they focus on that meaning, it puts them into a state—a hypnotic state of inward focus. When they focus on the meaning that they give to our statement for that moment, they enter trance.

In this text, a hypnotic state or trance refers to a focusing of attention on a thought, idea, concept, thing, etc. which excludes all other focusing on anything else. Now, as we focus on just one chunk of data, we are able to move or transport that chunk to another. In effect, we take the first thought and apply it to another thought.

For instance, if I have a problem and, during hypnosis, my focus moves from my problem to focusing on a resource for healing my problem, I can so focus on the resource that I realize its ability to solve my problem. Then, I can move that resource to the problem and solve my problem by putting new meaning to the problem (Meta-stating). The process resembles using a computer to put up a picture of a person's face on the screen and then 'try on' different hairstyles or colors. In hypnosis you can take the problem to the infinite collection of possibilities and select the one that works for you.

The content of the problem becomes open to change from the new information that exists in our memories or imagination. This information resides in the unconscious mind. Trance permits taking conscious mind material (the problem in this example), cut off from the unconscious mind, and integrating it with the rich resources of the unconscious mind (the resource). To distinguish conscious from unconscious mind you could think of your conscious mind as represented by where you are physically, right now, as you read this. Your unconscious mind is everywhere else in the universe. And since your response to this statement is a trance, just imagine the possibilities.

Chapter One

The Conscious–Unconscious Mind Split

This book explores the function of three particular factors that allow the mind to be susceptible to hypnotic language. These three factors are the *conscious–unconscious mind split*, the *cognitive style* of processing information that we rely on during our childhood years and the *perceptual principles of Gestalt psychology*. After describing these concepts and their dynamics, we will explain the role they each play in generating hypnotic language. This will allow us to identify and understand the construction, purpose and effect of hypnotic language.

The bulk of the text consists of hypnotic language patterns that will illustrate these three principles. We will explain the logic and purpose of these language patterns. Additionally, case examples will show the application and effect of these language patterns. Hypnotic language rarely provides the entire solution to a client's problem; rather it may provide a sort of linguistic loosening or tightening device. This means that in the process of arriving at a solution, hypnotic language provides this loosening device that allows the client to release rigid thoughts, emotions or behaviors.

> **Hypnotic language rarely provides the entire solution to a client's problem; rather it may provide a sort of linguistic loosening or tightening device.**

Hypnotic language may also provide the final tightening after a mental, emotional or behavioral shift to hold the change in place. And certainly, at times, hypnotic language may truly stimulate the full change process. This now leads to identifying and explaining the concept of hypnotic language through the three facets that allow the mind to be susceptible to hypnotic language.

The Conscious–Unconscious Mind Split

Most forms of communication create a trance. It happens when we develop an exclusive focus on the message that the communicator is sending to the receiver. Communication occurs through any one of the five senses alone, or in combination.

Consider the chef who creates a collection of flavors and textures for your palate. If prepared properly, you will lapse into a trance filled with delight over the flavors, texture and other aspects of the culinary masterpiece. You will want more and will probably return to that restaurant. Even the invitation to partake in the gustatory trance involves trance through the visual and olfactory and, at times, auditory senses. The foods you choose and the style of foods you prefer come to be so, in part, because the chef succeeded in 'trancing' or entrancing you. Of course, while in this trance you will decide if the experience is satisfying enough for you to want to repeat it in the future. But a trance must happen before you determine the quality of the experience.

The way all communication involves trance holds true for your other senses. Consider having a massage from a masseuse. The pathway to the intended relief travels through a trance state. You miss the message of the massage if your mind wanders from the physical sensations to some task in your past or future. One of the reasons some people buy the clothes they wear is because of the way the clothes feel on their skin (kinesthetic buyers). Before purchasing they will feel the material with their fingers and evaluate if the fabric feels right to them. This evaluation involves a light trance as this person focuses on the 'feel' of the material and then imagines what it will feel like when they wear that piece of clothing.

Music easily induces an auditory trance-state. The musician's ability to induce a trance through music determines whether or not the listener accepts the music. Music-induced trance makes for one of the most popular and easily accessed kinds of trances. Lovers of music spend millions of dollars each year buying music just because it induces an enjoyable trance within them. There are even certain sounds that induce a trance and pre-determined response. Various bells, whistles and sirens automatically activate a certain response. Some research indicates that various types of background music can encourage a person to buy more in a store or to eat more in a restaurant than normal.

Think about trances induced through the olfactory (smell) sense. Remember the enticing scent of a perfume or cologne. Or recall the emotionally warming aroma of bread baking. What about the concept of aromatherapy? This treatment banks on the trance inducing ability of scents for improving health and well-being. Scents for the sense to make cents, how do all those words I sent to you sound?

> **Scents for the sense to make cents,**
> **how do all these words I sent to you sound?**

Certainly we do not want to overlook trance induced through visual means. The visual artist, whether painter in any medium, sketch artist or photographer seeks to induce a trance by getting the attention of those who view her work. Go into an art gallery and watch the intense observers go into trance. If the visual aid propels you into a trance and in this trance your experience appeals to your emotions, you may buy the work of art. And what is very often the first catalyst of attraction between two eventually romantically involved people? Before you meet someone, what you see and then think provides the motivation for getting to know this person.

No doubt you can think of many other examples of how communication through the senses produces a trance in the receiver. If effective, the receiver of the communication goes into a trance. Consider these questions:

- What features make some communication more effective than other communication for inducing a trance?

- What makes the receiver of linguistic communication respond to the invitation and go into trance?

- What takes place while one is in trance that makes this form of communication produce change in the receiver?

9

> **Hypnotic language presupposes a conscious mind and a rich resource filled unconscious mind.**

To answer these questions we first explore the mental ingredients that play a role in hypnotic trance. Hypnotic language presupposes a conscious mind and a rich resource-filled unconscious mind. Another way of viewing the 'split-mind' involves what I refer to as *primary and secondary awareness*.

Primary awareness (the conscious mind) consists of your current awareness, in any given moment, your conscious mind. For instance, you are focusing on the words on this page right now. This is primary awareness. *Secondary awareness* (the unconscious mind) consists of all the other information you have gathered throughout your life, but do not presently realize in your primary awareness. Secondary awareness refers to the storehouse of information residing in your unconscious mind. You probably were not aware of your right big toe until these words just now called attention to it. Well, your unconscious mind or your secondary awareness knew about it all the time. You just weren't aware of it consciously.

> **George Miller (1956) determined the nine value upper limit of your primary awareness. His studies indicated that we can consciously hold 7±2 items in awareness at any given moment of time.**

George Miller (1956) determined the nine value upper limit of your primary awareness. His studies indicated that we consciously hold 7±2 items in awareness at any given moment of time. Yet, it would appear that we experience subtle 'knowings' that 'all other information' resides within. For example, you may get a 'gut feeling' that something's wrong like leaving a stove burner on after leaving your house. You don't know just what is specifically wrong but you trust this 'instinct' and return home to check the stove.

> **We believe that hypnotic language overwhelms our primary awareness limitations in order to communicate with our secondary awareness.**

We believe that hypnotic language overwhelms our primary awareness limitations in order to communicate with our secondary awareness. Secondary awareness represents everything not of primary awareness or everything other than your awareness now. Secondary awareness has knowledge of the complete resource inventory within your conscious and unconscious mind. The style and content of hypnotic language invites your primary awareness to focus upon the content of the spoken words, but then the content exceeds the processing ability of the primary awareness. This results in passing the information to the secondary awareness where everything becomes possible.

The Thalamus and Cortex

Further, it seems that the thalamus and cortex play a role in this primary and secondary awareness. While likely remaining unproven, I will present this position for your consideration. Alfred Korzybski took this position in his class work that initiated the field of general semantics, *Science and Sanity* (1994 [1941]).

The thalamus serves the role of initial processing site for all incoming sensory information with the exception of the sense of smell— Korzybski's lower abstraction level.

Some say the sense of smell can trigger a memory faster than the other senses. Perhaps this bypassing of the thalamus is the reason for this. This is an established fact in neurology, as noted by both Bandler and Grinder, in *The Structure of Magic* and Korzybski in *Science and Sanity*. After the other senses pass information to the thalamus for general identifying and categorizing, the thalamus then passes the sensory information to various lobes of the cortex for more detailed analysis and complex meaning making.

> **Support for the role of the thalamus and cortex in simple and complex processing of stimuli comes, in part, from the work of Jean Piaget (1965).**

Support for the role of the thalamus and cortex in simple and complex processing of stimuli comes, in part, from the work of Jean Piaget (1965). Piaget studied the cognitive development of many hundreds of children of various ages. His research spanned several decades. One way Piaget studied children's cognitive development involved observing their ability to process and understand information of varying degrees of complexity. Piaget presented children of different ages with a reasoning problem. He observed how the children understood the variables within the problem and how they manipulated the information to reach their conclusion.

For example, Piaget would show children a photo of two trees. The two trees differed in type and height. Piaget then asked children of different ages which tree was older. Invariably, children below the age of seven, or thereabouts, chose the taller tree as the older. Children older than about seven years of age asked when the trees were planted to find out the age of the trees. The older children had the ability to take more information into account for reasoning. They could do more complex thinking involving simultaneous consideration of different categories of information. The children over seven years of age not only looked at the height of the trees but thought about additional factors that may account for the difference in height. They did this through the higher level (Meta-level) processes of the cerebral cortex.

Data Categories of Complexity

We list here the four different categories of data that represent ever-increasing degrees of mental/cognitive complexity (the capacity of processing more and more complex abstractions—meta-level processes). These categories are *nominal, ordinal, interval* and *ratio*.

Nominal data represents itself in all-or-nothing terms. When you place any information within a category or give it a general label it becomes nominal data. Information fitting into this data level includes: winning–losing, pregnant–not pregnant, good–bad, etc. This level of data contains no gray area. Nominal data also evidences itself when a person speaks in all-or-nothing language patterns, i.e. 'You are either with me or against me'. Some information naturally lends itself to fitting as nominal data (pregnant or not pregnant) and sometimes people force-fit data into the nominal category by ignoring the shades of gray, i.e. 'You are either with me or against me'.

This nominal perceptual style (way of processing information), or Meta-program in Neuro-Linguistic Programming (NLP), limits awareness and choice (see Hall and Bodenhamer, *Figuring Out People*, 1997a). This type of thinking frequently accompanies limiting beliefs and their consequences. Young children cannot escape this style of thinking due to their cognitive limitations. They cannot simultaneously hold differing or competing ideas so their evaluations of situations become either–or types. When under stress some adults revert to the child-like either–or thinking style.

This style of thinking may also occur in adults when they feel emotional stress. Information within nominal data fits in one of two groups. The information is dichotomized into either–or categories. The details either don't exist, such as when a woman is pregnant or not pregnant, or they get left out of the evaluation. This leaving out of details is one of the trademarks of personality disordered people. In particular, borderline personalities do a process that is called affective splitting. These people either hate someone or love someone. No middle ground exists. Another example could be someone believing that someone is all good or all bad with no in-between. Reframing as a therapeutic tool relies on this nominal category because it seeks to change the meaning of a circumstance. In doing this, it shifts the meaning from one category to another more resourceful category of meaning. For example, just because you changed some behavior and now someone objects doesn't mean you have to return to your former ways. It actually means you have successfully changed and that you can now more fully strengthen this new way, reaping the benefits.

Watzlawick, Weakland and Fisch (1974) talk about reframing in these terms:

> In its most abstract terms, reframing means changing the emphasis from one class membership of an object to another, equally valid class membership, or, especially, introducing such a new class membership into the conceptualization of all concerned. (p. 98)

Watzlawick *et al.* (1974) emphasized three aspects related to reframing. They state that our experience of the world is based on categorization of the objects we perceive into classes. The authors also state that once an object is conceptualized as the member of a given class, it is extremely difficult to see it as belonging also to another class. This class membership of an object is called its 'reality'. Thus, anybody who sees it as the member of another class must be mad or bad.

Once an object is conceptualized as the member of a given class, it is extremely difficult to see it as belonging also to another class. This class membership of an object is called its 'reality.'

Finally, what makes reframing such an effective tool of change involves frame stability. That is, once we perceive the alternative class membership(s), we cannot so easily go back to the trap and the anguish of a former view of 'reality.'

The second category for evaluating the complexity of mental processing ability is that of *ordinal data*. Ordinal data provide a way of ranking the complexity of information in terms of the increasing or decreasing of some quality within the data. Ordinal data compare stimuli and generate an order or rank using relative comparisons from within the group.

As an example, when children run a race they receive recognition in terms of where they are placed at the finish. Ordinal data reveal which child ran faster than another child, though all the children ran. The child finishing second is not twice as fast as the child finishing fourth. The positions contain no flexibility or degrees.

Positions exist, but not on a sliding scale. Within ordinal data no true zero exists because the data represent comparisons within the group rather than comparisons to an entity outside the group. All data in the group possess some degree of the quality measured, so results are relative. Within individuals, emotional states may receive ranking in terms of being stronger or more intense than other states on a continuum. For one person, anxiety may rank as a stronger state than worry and worry more intense than concern. Or a person may say that they feel more scared than angry about his child being very late coming home one evening.

Interval data include the characteristics of the first two categories and adds more sophistication through more abstraction. Not only do the items within interval data relate to each other in terms of rank, but they also vary in degrees of a relationship with each other. The interval between items has meaning. The details receive attention and become important in evaluating the data. Ranking children who run a race represents ordinal data. But if these children's race times get included along with their order of finish then interval data occurs. In this case, the race times serve at a Meta-level to the ordinal data (Hall, 1995, 1996, 1997).

In these usages, the term 'Meta' simply means 'above' or 'beyond'. The structure of Meta-states naturally organizes them in an ordinal data way. Each higher Meta-state controls the state below it so a sort of built-in ranking happens with Meta-states.

In the Meta-states® model, Hall has drawn upon the work of Alfred Korzybski (*Science and Sanity*, 1933/1994) and Gregory Bateson (*Steps to an Ecology of Mind*, 1972). This has led to an understanding of how our brains not only have thoughts about our immediate experiences of the outside world (primary level thoughts) but also thoughts about thoughts (Meta-level thoughts, or Meta-cognition feelings about feelings [Meta-feelings], etc.). Bateson revealed that when we take one thought and then create another thought about that thought, the original thought will experience some modification from the second and higher-level thought. Bateson said higher-level thoughts, i.e. thoughts about thoughts, modulate (change) lower-level thoughts.

For example, I can experience fear about some external experience. From that I will have a certain state of mind. Now, if I become fearful of my fear, what then happens? My fear will intensify. But what if I become calm about my fear? What will then happen? I will certainly experience a different state of mind when I bring fear to bear on fear. Try it out. Think of something that you have some fear about. Now, access a state of calmness and bring calmness to bear on the fear. What happens?

Back to our example with interval data. When a competitor who finishes a race looks at his own placement and then 'brings to bear' the collective individual times on his placement in the race, a more complex relationship develops. He Meta-states his individual placement by bringing the other individual times to bear on his placement. This process can drastically change the original thought-feelings he had about his placement. If a racer finishes a race in third place, but in the process broke his personal time record that would certainly change his thought-feelings about being placed third and not first.

How much time did the first place runner finish ahead of the second- or third-place finishers? All of this information 'brought to bear' on the time finishes will modulate or change his perception of his finish. These comparisons can also occur between any of the items within the category. Time itself represents interval data. Ten seconds is twice as much time as five seconds and 15 minutes is half as much time as 30 minutes. When a child begins to abstract and have thoughts about thoughts, they have begun to process interval data.

The interval level of data permits hypnotic induction for comparing different data which requires a 'going inside' which in turn creates trance.

As a side note, did you find that this interval level of data permits hypnotic induction? Did you go into a light trance when you compared the larger time increment with the smaller and then the smaller with the larger, essentially a switching of perspectives (a going Meta through having thoughts about thoughts)?

The comparison of seconds and minutes went in two directions and involved degrees of difference. Two computations take place at the same time, rank and degree of difference. Prior to this level of data only one computation occurs, either–or or rank order. With interval data degree of difference become perceivable making the continuum more detailed. The interval level of data permits hypnotic induction for comparing different data which requires a 'going inside' which in turn creates trance. It is important to remember that in hypnosis, any statement or question that requires a person to 'go inside', to respond or to answer will induce trance.

Ratio data make up the most sophisticated type of data. While interval data possess a zero point such as with time and weight, the zero holds no meaning beyond an absence of quantity. Zero represents a void with no measurement below it. You cannot experience 'below an absence of time' nor can weight measure below an absence, so we must restrict these to interval data. On the other hand, the data in the ratio category contain the characteristics of the previous three categories and add another dimension. Interrelationships between data occur, but a zero point receives meaning rather than representing just an absence.

Our number system represents ratio data. This category of data possesses a zero point but this zero holds actual meaning within a larger continuum. The zero in our number system can play an influential role in relating to the other data within the group. The later two data categories possess significantly more sophistication. They move beyond just all-or-nothing labels and simple rankings to degrees of relations between data and finally to an infinite continuum. This last category permits awareness of and access to the realm of all possibilities within each of us, as we possess an infinite continuum. Our brains can have thoughts about thoughts ad infinitum.

To illustrate all four data categories in action, consider an example of conflict resolution. Labeling the situation as 'conflict' reflects nominal data. Ordinal data come into effect because the people in the conflict each hold a different rank order of importance about the issue in conflict. Otherwise, no conflict could exist since they would be in agreement about the issue. Interval data occur in the value attributed to the various agreement possibilities. In the process of attempting to reach a compromise each side may receive various concessions. These concessions and their various values hopefully add up to what both sides believe is equal. The concessions take the form of interval data because they exist in various amounts and the difference between them has significance. This method of various concessions for each side can bring a solution to a conflict.

Ratio data emerge when a person rises to a higher level of thinking (a Meta-level) that permits seeing all possibilities in no longer pre-arranged or set styles. In rising to this higher level, we in fact 'step outside' the system and from a Meta-position view ourselves within the context of the entire system. By stepping outside our selves and the system (conceptual dissociation) we remove ourselves from much of the emotion and operate from a more rational perspective.

> **By going Meta, the world becomes denominalized (or unfrozen) and all things become possible. This allows new and creative solutions to challenges to arise; even the concept of conflict disappears here.**

From that Meta-level or 'system's position', new creative arrangements now become available to us. We can see how each part in the system functions in relation to the other parts. Since we have 'stepped outside' the system and ourselves we invite our unconscious mind to access additional resources. When we are in the conflict, we feel it intensely. And, in feeling it intensely we tend to operate off our emotions rather than our intuition thus shutting down many of our unconscious resources. By going Meta, the world becomes denominalized (or unfrozen) and all things become possible. This allows new and creative solutions to challenges to arise; even the concept of conflict disappears here.

Our ability to think in terms of these various data categories develop over time as a matter of development or maturity. In the process of human cognitive development, as chronicled by Piaget, children gain the ability to process data on a more complex level after the age of seven and increase this ability until maximal development around age 11–12. The thalamus seems to remain generally steady in presence and capacity throughout development. The changes apparently occur within the regions of the cortex, the complex data processing center. By this logic, we suspect that the thalamus accounts for lower level functions such as nominal and ordinal data. This then passes the role of more complex processing, interval and ratio data (Meta-level thinking), to the cortex as it develops this ability over the course of child development. The end result is that the structure of hypnotic language invokes the more sophisticated capacities of the cortex for understanding the message. And this development seems to occur after the age of seven up to age 11–12.

The structure of hypnotic language invokes the more sophisticated capacities of the cortex for understanding the message. And this development seems to occur after the age of seven up to age 11–12.

Later, in examining the thought patterns of children under the age of 11, you will find that almost all, if not all, limiting beliefs and states develop out of limited cognitive capacity. This means that, given the child's brain and maturity development, the early mapping reflected the best the child could do. And yet, it also reflects the thinking level and skills of a *child*, not of a mature mind.

The point of therapy in general, and hypnotic language in particular, involves transporting the complex thought skills back in time allowing this ability to reprocess 'the limiting cognitive knot' in the persons' psyche. This means that you can use what you know now on what you did not know then. You can update your old maps and create new and better referent experiences.

Nominal and ordinal data, or perceptual styles, can then become interval and ratio. This allows more details to come to light, popping the Gestalt bubble and freeing the person from her previous restrictions. An issue gets shifted from the conscious mind's limited thinking ability to the unconscious mind's unlimited thinking ability.

Chapter Two
Cognitive Factors in Hypnotic Language

Anytime you concentrate on any stimuli, you go into a trance for at least a brief time to perceive, encode and store the information. Since this is the process of storing then it also needs to be the process of accessing and altering the stored information.

The next category of factors contributing to hypnotic language's effectiveness involves the specific cognitive style of processing information. When unconscious parts form or limiting beliefs originate, they result from the brain operating in certain ways (more on beliefs in chapter 4). These parts, or limitations, require particular perception and thought in order to generate and remain supported. Anytime you pay attention to any stimuli you must go into a trance for at least a brief time to perceive, encode and store the information. Since this is the process of storing, then it also needs to be the process of accessing and altering the stored information. As an analogy, if you plan to change the shape of ice, first melt it, then decide what mold you want for the final shape, fill the mold with the water and refreeze it.

> **Hypnotic language returns the mind to the scene of the crime in a general way. It thaws the belief or state.**

In a general way, hypnotic language returns the mind to the scene of the crime. It thaws the belief or state. When beliefs or concepts become rigid, they reach a condition known as nominalized. The word 'educating' nominalizes into 'education'. 'Depressing' nominalizes into 'depression'. In general, nominalizing converts a process into a rigid, frozen condition. Hypnotic language comes in a non-traditional form of language so it denominalizes, or de-crystallizes a concept or belief. The hypnotic language itself comes in a denominalized form within the general guidelines of language. To comprehend the language you must dissociate (step outside of, go Meta to) from the rigid nominalized state and associate (be totally present in) into a denominalized state. So just listening or reading and processing hypnotic language dissociates you (a Meta-state) from your present, now former state. Then you can deal with specific content or states with free choice.

> **Actually, all effective therapy seems to involve hypnotherapy.**

The client must associate into the problem state then dissociate from it, access a resource state, associate into it and apply this new resource to the problem state. John Overdurf taught me (BB) what he calls 'The Mother of All NLP'. I have found his model most helpful and, in my opinion, true to fact. He suggests that all NLP patterns that work will consist of four basic steps. I believe that effective hypnosis follows the same patterns.

1. First the client must associate into the problem state. Most of the time clients are associated into the problem state when they arrive in your office.

2. Second, the hypnotherapist dissociates the client from his problem. This conceptually moves the client to a position Meta to the problem. From a dissociative perspective, the client can see himself within the context of the problem but outside of it. This position allows for the consideration of other alternatives. You cannot solve a problem on the level of the problem. Dissociating moves the client Meta to the problem.

3. Third, from the dissociated perspective, the hypnotherapist directs the client to discover a resource state, associate into it and apply this new resource to the problem state (Meta-stating). It is at this point that the efficient hypnotherapist becomes a Meta-stating genius. Richard Bandler offers a superb example of skill in this area.

4. Finally, the hypnotherapist Future Paces the client with the additional resources. NLP future pacing is a Meta-stating process as the hypnotherapist takes the client with his resources and applies (Meta-states) these to future occurrences. Before the therapy the client would run the old

problem state in any perceived future memories but now, with the new resources, the client runs the resource state as he brings it to bear on future-oriented perceptions.

Actually, all effective therapy seems to involve hypnotherapy. Unless you and the client focus exclusively on the issue, a trance, then no real change can happen. No matter the model used in accomplishing 'The Mother of All NLP', hypnosis will be involved. Sometimes the process occurs overtly; at other times the induction is covert. Either way, or with any style of therapy, hypnotherapy takes place in the process of change. Hypnotic language represents one of the more direct ways of accessing the seat of change.

For change to happen in therapy, the client must first associate into the problem state. The client then dissociates from it, accesses and associates into a resource state, and applies this resource to the problem state. Sometimes the process occurs overtly, while sometimes the induction is less obvious. But either way, or with any style of therapy, hypnotherapy takes place in the process of change. Hypnotic language represents one of the more direct ways of accessing the seat of change.

> **More specifically, hypnotic language communicates with the brain in the same language and cognitive style that goes on while forming the problem state or belief.**

More specifically, hypnotic language communicates with the brain in the same language and cognitive style that is used while forming the problem state or belief. Almost all, if not all, limiting beliefs about self, others or life form during childhood. By childhood, I mean the first 12–15 years of life.

Communicating with the mind in the way it thought during the formation of the limiting beliefs allows access to, and altering of, the contents of the 'problem'. Hypnotic language speaks the language that was spoken when the problem formed. Thus, accessing and altering the problem becomes available. If these beliefs or states form in adulthood they still conform to certai laws of misperception—flawed laws you may call them.

Certain perceptual flaws must occur to form a limiting belief or non-resource state. These flaws dominate childhood perception and also take place when developing a 'problem state' in adulthood (Burton, 1999). These perceptual flaws of childhood, to be explained shortly, include:

1. *Either-or thinking*. Thinking in black and white terms, all or nothing. (We have discussed this earlier when we considered the nominal category of the data categories of complexity).

2. *Irreversibility*. Inability to perceive events as they existed before the trauma.

3. *Over-generalizing*. Using inductive reasoning to draw conclusions and generalize the conclusion. This is a sort of Meta-level inductive reasoning.

4. *Egocentrism*. A focusing on self to the exclusion of other points of view.

5. *Transductive logic*. Two events occurring closely in time receive cause–effect attributes.

6. *Centering*. Focusing on only one element of a whole, excluding other important details.

7. *Inductive logic*. Reasoning from a specific event and making general inferences.

8. *Animism*. Giving inanimate objects life. To a child, 'Teddy Bear' is alive and the walls can hear.

The brain utilizes these styles of thinking when forming the limiting belief or problem state in the first place. Hypnotic language also assumes the brain will use these cognitive styles when the hypnotherapist delivers the hypnotic language. And, since the brain utilized these thinking styles in formulating the problem to begin with, when the neurology of the problem is re-introduced to the same type of thinking in the hypnotic language patterns the hypnotherapist will have instant rapport with the problem. This happens because the problem-state will have familiarity with the hypnotic linguistic structure as it activates and conforms to the structure of the problem.

> **The purpose of therapy is to give old behaviors new choices for obtaining their outcome.**

The reframing, or healing, of the problem happens as the linguistic structure of the problem-state is given new and healthier choices for obtaining its original purpose. NLP asserts that all behaviors have behind them a positive intent for the person doing the behavior. Old thinking patterns that developed during the earlier years of life when we had limited resources often fail to serve us in adult life. The purpose of therapy is to give these old behaviors new choices for obtaining their outcome.

We can utilize similar linguistic structures through hypnotic language patterns in accessing those old and limited thinking patterns and give them new choices. By giving them new choices we bring a familiar linguistically structured resource to bear on the problem. Once in place, the new perspective will take center stage and direct the individual to more constructive ways of thinking, feeling and behaving.

Hypnotic language speaks with most of the same characteristics as the perceptual flaws that form the 'problem'. These perceptual flaws include *all or nothing thinking*. It is either black or white; there is no gray area. This shows up within the double-bind pattern.

Hypnotic language often uses *animism* referring to inanimate objects as though they possess human qualities. Animism is another of the traits of childhood thinking. Animism occurs when inanimate objects are given animate qualities. All objects come alive when animism is at play or work. This means that, to a child, the walls do have ears and the shoes under their bed can come to life. Their teddy bear or doll is a real living and breathing being. The shirt in the closet becomes a monster in the night. Cartoons, animated films and children's books utilize this animism principle to reach children where they think. All of us retain this ability throughout our life. We just put so many layers over it (Meta-states), but it still resides within.

The hypnotic language category of selectional restriction violation draws on this mental skill and harks the listener back to his childhood. Now the root of the limiting belief becomes accessible because the listener associates into his childhood mentality. A person never seems to lose this ability. At most they just place other layers of alternate thinking styles over it.

Irreversibility refers to the inability to remember how things were before the present set of circumstances. When a person is associated into a state it is usually hard for them to remember what they thought or felt before the current state. To assist them in remembering, we need to dissociate them from their current state. Hypnotic language helps a person with limiting beliefs to dissociate and remember how they were before the limitations. When associated into their new resource state, they will often find irreversibility happens again. Since they are associated into a resource state they really won't care to remember their old limitations.

Over-generalizing happens when a person jumps to conclusions based on limited information. They will notice one piece of a current situation that resembles a previous one and assume they must be the *same*. This makes up prejudice. The limited awareness of childhood, and often of primary states, results in over-generalizing. The details of a circumstance get ignored because the mind does not consider the differences; instead, it only notices the similarities.

Egocentricity describes yet another quality present in all children. And it shows up in many of the hypnotic language patterns. The egocentric person focuses on self to the exclusion of other points of view. Egocentricity involves an individual believing that their point of view exists as the only point of view thus all others think the same way. The egocentric assumes that their own map of the world governs the thinking that occurs in everyone's head. Hypnotic language requests an exclusive focus on self and this request occurs in several patterns. Egocentric thought acts as the undercurrent in all hypnotic language as it requests the listener to utilize this skill for application to self.

Children use *transductive logic* in explaining events in their world. Children tend to take one specific event and generalize from that specific event. A classic example is of the mother in San Francisco who told her child that if he slammed the door, something terrible would happen. Well, he slammed the door and they had a severe earthquake. Unable to go 'Meta' to the experience, the child believed his bad behavior 'caused' the earthquake. Don't you wish you had that kind of power? A child's mind does.

This type of thinking leads children to conclude that events coinciding in time serve as acceptable explanations for causal agents. The family dog walks into the room just when the child spills his milk. Using transductive logic, the child attributes the spill to the dog. It seems all of us at any age seek knowing cause. In the primitive thinking patterns of children seeking a 'cause' feels like it saves them from taking responsibility for their own behaviors.

Asking the 'why' question so often seeks for justification for doing the behavior and rarely leads to solving the behavior (See Dennis and Jennifer Chong, *Don't Ask Why?! A Book about the Structure of Blame, Bad Communication and Miscommunication*, 1991). Asking 'why?' shifts our perspective to the past. Yet we will not find the solution in the past. The solution exists in present mental constructions. No wonder asking why leads to the frustration of unsatisfactory solutions.

The Anatomy of a Problem (From *States of Equilibrium* by John Burton, forthcoming)

Piaget's meticulous mapping of these cognitive principles and their function, contributes considerably to understanding how people function, or dysfunction. It may be safe to say that these cognitive styles or Meta-programs that develop in childhood during the first seven years of life, make up the basic ingredients of most, if not all, problem states. It may be safe to say that these cognitive styles or Meta-programs that develop during the first seven years of life make up the basic ingredients of most, if not all, problem states.

Consider the primary state of anger as an example. Anger carries with it impulsive urges much like early childhood developmental stages identified in children. Anger as a primary state exemplifies *generalizing* (how quickly do you believe the offending person always does this or everyone treats you this way?). If you generalize like this and believe either one, then anger intensifies. If you do not use this generalization then anger decreases.

Centration displays itself when anger and the 'offending' event become the sole focus, excluding contrary evidence. You dwell on the other's 'offending' act to the exclusion of all that is contrary. You may then go on a hunt for other similar examples from this person's past. Irreversibility leads you to further dwelling and loss of memory for the state or person's behavior prior to the adverse event. You lose awareness of resourceful states to respond from and find it increasingly difficult to focus on anything but the upsetting event. In fact, if you consider contrary evidence, your anger modifies into another state such as confusion or curiosity about the event, becoming solution-oriented instead of self-protecting and vengeful.

Transductive reasoning comes into play when you believe the other person's behavior caused your emotional state. You notice your anger came right after the other person behaved a certain way or said certain words. You attribute your anger to the other person because that was the event just before your anger started. Never mind what took place in your mind that really generated the anger. Anger and its Meta-programs prevent considering other sources of anger, other points of view or additional information outside the initial perception.

The cognitive styles identified by Piaget build walls around information and beliefs that prevent alternative information from being considered.

We use these same cognitively limited styles when we generate problem states or limiting beliefs. If you alter one of the perceptual pieces the whole irrational structure crumbles. The cognitive styles identified by Piaget build walls around information and beliefs that prevent alternative information from being considered. Therapy in general, and hypnotic language in particular, challenges the narrow thoughts or beliefs and expands awareness. This expanded awareness defeats and removes these cognitive clogs.

Hypnotic Language

Hypnotic language plays to this need to know 'why' in several ways. When a person leaves behind former meanings attached to familiar items in her world, she can frequently only tolerate this for a short time. The passion for explanations drives this cognitive hunger. And so she becomes mentally hungry for meaning and structure.

For the therapist this opens up the opportunity to supply new possibilities that the client can use to explain and 'cause' new outcomes. At some level the client seeks a tool that can cause her desired outcome. In hypnosis the client is more receptive to using new tools. The client can also form new mental associations or structure in her mind. This makes for new belief systems and new sources of believed cause.

By the concept of centering we refer to the process of a person focusing her attention on a narrow range of information. That excludes other significant information about the stimuli or event. In practice, centering equates to trance. While in trance a person focuses intently on one small area. Likewise, in centering, the focus of the person narrows to a fine point to the exclusion of all other details. In centering, the person takes some portion of an event or stimulus out of context. Children remain in this centering state for about the first seven years of their life producing quite an effective learning machine due to their intense focus. While effective for learning, the limited information available through the narrow focus may produce significantly limiting beliefs.

Hypnotic language relies on centering to induce a trance, but then leads the focus to something other than the limiting belief and event, i.e. the resource for healing. Hypnosis allows the client to be shown an alternative resource on which to center and then consider the benefits of this new resource in his life. In essence, the trance allows the client to choose between focusing on the problem or focusing on the resource. In either case, the centering process takes place. Focusing on the resource just makes constructive use of the already existing centering.

> **Hypnotic language relies on centering to induce a trance, but then leads the focus to something other than the limiting belief and event, i.e. the resource for healing.**

A particular case serves as a good example to illustrate the influence of these cognitive principles and how hypnotic language can bring about a more effective choice. This case involved Doug who tended to fly into a rage when others made comments that he perceived questioned his sense of personal worth. Doug and his fiancée, Linda, came in for counseling. Doug's temper outbursts had almost ended their relationship. Doug regularly took offense at benign comments that Linda made about his actions and his appearance. Both agreed, when looking back, that the comments could easily have been taken as either lightweight or offering alternative perspectives rather than criticism. But when Doug heard Linda's criticism, he immediately personalized them as a threat to his sense of personal worth. Upon hearing her comments, Doug would go into a rage. He would yell, cuss and berate Linda. This led to several short break-ups between them. In order for their marriage to survive, they had to overcome these accumulated hurdles.

Several cognitive elements became evident when Doug described his reasoning about these comments that led to rage.

First, Doug took them as personal (*egocentrism*). Doug believed that Linda's comments must be about him. Doug had 'I' trouble as his awareness totally focused on himself. Rather than being comments about a behavior or his appearance, Doug felt the comments referred to him as a person thus addressing his sense of personal worth. He ignored the lengthy relationship history with his fiancée that included much mutual support and encouragement (irreversibility).

Doug admitted that the good times occupied at least 98% of their time together. The fits of rage required *centering* his focus on the 2% of the time with 'derogatory' comments. Centering on these comments led Doug to conclude, 'She is always finding fault with me'. So, in Doug's eyes, Linda 'caused' his rage (*transductive logic*). The rage response also required *over-generalizing and black-white thinking*. Due to Doug's tendency to center his focus on just the bad times with Linda, he over-generalized to 'all' of their relationship as being bad. Nor, could Doug see any shades of good or bad. In his mind it was either good or bad, and mostly bad. He *inductive-ly* reasoned that since he perceived Linda as making specific judgments about his sense of personal worth, she must have believed that everything about him had a bad connotation in her eyes (*Inductive logic*). Egocentrism prevented Doug from taking Linda's point of view. Doug could not consider a different purpose for the comments at the time they were spoken.

The first goal of the intervention involved expanding their aware-ness and thus opening them up to additional information. Accomplishing this goal involved injecting broader awareness into the cognitive cluster that generated the rage. I first mentioned to Doug the possibility that much more was going on between him and Linda than he had previously noticed. When he agreed that this was a possibility, I invited his curiosity about what was going on outside his centering focus. I further suggested that if he did find different information and interpretations, the conflict might disappear and that this disappearing conflict could allow him to feel better. This comment appealed to his egocentricity.

Then I left him wondering by suggesting that he might never know what existed outside his point of view, which possibly excluded the most helpful information, the very information that could make the problem disappear. And just how would he ever know? This suggested the possibility that his perception was incomplete and tended to place in him a desire to search for com-pleteness. This linguistic structure is a Gestalt perceptual principle known as closure. We will explore this model later in more detail. Closure provided a motivation for Doug to learn more.

The following recounts the hypnotic language pattern I used with Doug:

> I realize that you deeply want to make your mark in this world and that this means a lot to you. I also realize that you have a sense of urgency about this so you may at times want to move too quickly without enough information. This leads you to feel frustrated and angry instead of the mark you want to make more deeply. And so perhaps a different mark, Doug,

not to confuse names because you know you really are Doug, but consider what kind of mark you can make when your confusion leads you to place a question mark, Doug, between you and the information around you. Keeping this mark in place can allow you to explore more and find more making a deeper mark because of your question mark, Doug, in between you and the world, you see, more information as your question leads to expanding what you know. This then leads you to more effective choices now, won't it?

Following this pattern Doug noticed that he actually visualized a question mark superimposed on his external world. He then noticed how this encouraged him to ask questions of others. The question mark served as a reminder to him to collect more information rather than jumping to conclusions from a limited amount of information as he had done with Linda. The placement of the question mark also reportedly worked very well to bring about his desired outcome—no more rage response. In a conversation with Doug six months later, he reported to me that the conflicts of the past had disappeared. In fact he and Linda had arranged to have their wedding in just two weeks.

Chapter Three

Gestalt Perceptual Principles in Hypnotic Language

In addition to the cognitive elements that make the brain conducive to hypnotic language, several principles of human perception play a role in making hypnotic language effective in changing perception. The perceptual principles identified by the field of Gestalt psychology play a crucial role in the process of hypnotic language.

Gestalt psychology traces its roots back to the late 1800s. It generally explores the process of human perception and the overall ebb and flow of interaction between the environment and a person. Gestalt psychology seeks to explain the process and structure of psychological events. In part, Gestalt psychology wants to reveal how people make sense of their surroundings and how they weave this understanding into an overall concept of their world.

In NLP terms, these perceptual principles make up Meta-programs (Hall and Bodenhamer, 1997a). These Meta-programs or perceptual filters provide the tools with which each person makes his map of the world. Early contributors to the research and body of knowledge in Gestalt psychology include Max Wertheimer, Wolfgang Kohler and Curt Koffka. Many others contributed to the foundation and superstructure. For the purpose of this book these three named contributors will serve as references.

The research of human perception reveals several principles about how a person organizes stimuli in his mind. These principles include ways of grouping information. Starting with the most general principle of Gestalt psychology, people organize the stimuli they sense. How we organize stimuli provides predictable avenues for hypnotic language to travel to its mark, the unconscious mind, and then to constructively influence the listener. Not only do we organize the information we sense, but also we each organize it in specific consistent styles. The perceptual principles affecting hypnotic language's efficacy include:

1. Figure–ground
2. Likeness or similarity
3. Closure
4. Simplicity
5. Dissonance reduction
6. Continuation

Max Wertheimer first identified these perceptual principles in 1912. The original principles did not include dissonance reduction. I added this principle, due to the significant influence it exerts on perception and beliefs. Leon Festinger identified the concept of cognitive dissonance in 1957. The identified categories of perception, except dissonance, began as principles of visual perception. These same principles apply to how a person organizes auditory stimuli, thus forming a foundation for beliefs, states of mind-emotion and behavior.

What you hear and selectively pay attention to and how you organize this collection into meaningful information greatly determines your way of being. Hypnotic language addresses the principles of organization and invites different perceptions of old stimuli. Hypnotic language offers new stimuli that may very well result in the individual re-organizing their beliefs in a way that better serves them.

> **One factor playing a role in giving hypnotic language effectiveness is our innate need to organize what we sense in such a way that allows us to understand the information.**

So, one factor playing a role in giving hypnotic language effectiveness is our innate need to organize what we sense in such a way that allows us to understand the information. Humans use this natural organizational drive to provide perception or meaning in their world. Hypnotic language takes advantage of this process in order to influence thinking. The person who speaks the hypnotic language can know that whatever they convey will be taken in by the receiver and the receiver will at least attempt to organize it and make sense of it.

> **The person who speaks the hypnotic language can know that whatever they convey will be taken in by the receiver and the receiver will at least attempt to organize it and make sense of it.**

To process information requires the listener to at least consider the contents of the message. For example, we do not believe a person can think about or speak about a state of mind without becoming aware of the contents of that state to some degree. The more details included in the description, the closer the person comes to associating into the state. And, notice that the more details that get included, the more the data move from nominal to ordinal to interval and ratio. This further suggests that details invite the unconscious mind into the situation or state. So, for example, you cannot suggest someone is paranoid without first stepping, to some degree, up to or into the state of paranoia yourself. How else did you determine that the other person's words and behavior added up to paranoia? The same holds true for the states of joy, euphoria or profound peace. You will find this presupposition frequently drawn on within the hypnotic language patterns. Humans seem to naturally or innately empathize. What happens after this sort of involuntary reflex is up to the individual.

As humans we seem to need some way of organizing the stimuli we sense. Sensing any stimuli takes the form of receiving rather generic information in which you detect certain general traits of any stimuli. In your visual sense, if your eyes sense a flat piece of wood about one inch thick, perhaps two feet by four feet in a rectangular shape, suspended above the ground by four cylindrical shaped wooden pieces, what would you call this? Your sensing provides the general information to your brain and then perception gives meaning to the general information. You perceive a 'table' as the result.

This organizing need occurs, in part, because this allows perceiving and ultimate meaning making by our brain. The thalamus and various parts of the cortex team up for perception. Now you can organize by using data from the item you attend to in your environment (primary awareness) as with the just cited example of a table.

But you can also use the concept of a table from your more general secondary awareness and find an item that satisfies the criteria. You could use the roof of your car or a bicycle seat to rest an item on, just as you can rest an item on a table. You could use the bicycle seat or car roof as support underneath a document for your signing. Do realize 'table' can come from external cues (primary awareness) or internal criteria (secondary awareness). This latter source makes for creative solutions by focusing on just how to generate the desired outcome. The process of utilizing secondary awareness resembles deductive logic, reasoning from general to specific. Perception and primary awareness relies on inductive logic, moving from specific to general. The primary awareness processes external specific stimuli, analyzes it and then fits it into general categories already existing in the secondary awareness.

Considertheselettersruntogether. Now you felt compelled to decode the letters in the previous collection, didn't you? You just can't help it.

Considertheselettersruntogether. Now you felt compelled to decode the letters in the previous collection, didn't you? You just can't help it. And you went into a light trance to do this decoding. So by identifying the naturally occurring mental processes you can know that the listener will at least make an effort to comprehend what you say to them.

Moving to specific concepts from Gestalt psychology, the concept of figure-ground plays a powerfully influential role in hypnotic language and general psychological make-up. The figure–ground process essentially divides stimuli into those you attend and those you don't. This figure–ground division places data into its most basic form, nominal. The stimuli attended become the figure or foreground.

The classic Gestalt example of the Old Hag/Young Woman Picture (Figure 3:1) powerfully illustrates the figure–ground shift that occurs in perception. Some parts of the stimuli collection are combined to create a figure. The remaining stimuli constitute the ground or background. The figure you perceive depends on which half you use for the figure and which takes the ground role.

Figure–ground

Figure 3:1
Young Woman/Old Hag

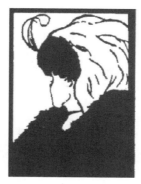

Michael Hall and I (BB) discuss this in our recently released book *The Structure of Excellence: Unmasking the Meta-Levels of 'Submodalities'* (1999):

> The classic gestalt example of *the Old Hag/Young Woman Picture* powerfully illustrates the foreground/background (figure/ground) shift that occurs in perception. Research experiments have even indicated that we can, apart from someone's consciousness, create a cognitive 'set' which can predispose a person to see one image rather than the other. Then, either by looking long enough or having someone suggest how they can see the other picture—one experiences *the gestalt shift.* Once that occurs, a person can generally shift back and forth at will. And yet even then, even though we fully know and believe that we can see each picture, we cannot see *both* images *simultaneously.* We can only see one or the other. It shifts digitally. Off. On.
>
> Something *attracts* us to 'see' the lines and shades in a certain way. Something *pulls us* toward *foregrounding* the 'young woman' or the 'old woman.' To look at one tiny line as a delicate eye lash, and a thicker line as a necklace, and another line to function as a beautiful jaw allows 'the young woman' to emerge from the picture. To see the same lines as the form of a large nose and the thicker line as a tightly pursed lips invites 'the old hag' image to emerge.

What we *foreground* thereby *sets the frame* so that the other pieces *organize* around, under, and in terms of that fore-ground. By so *foregrounding* certain elements and using them to construct certain meanings (semantic structures), a *configu-ration* arises that fits a form, image, and meaning that we *bring to the lines and shades.*

When a person cannot 'see' one emergent image, we some-times point with our finger and say, 'Just look at it this way.' 'Imagine that this line *is* an eye lash…' 'Now do you see it?' Having articulated the details that enable us to *configure* the gestalt (the overall systemic configuration), we can then begin to intentionally run *the Gestalt Switch.* We can fore-ground and background. With practice, we can do this in a split second until it seems that we can almost hold both images simultaneously.

To *highlight* one representation by necessity means that we *downplay* other representations. Frequently, such highlighting will even *hide* other ways of viewing things. Lakoff and Johnson (1980) describe this cognitive mechanism as inherent in 'categorization.' 'A categorization is a natural way of iden-tifying a *kind* of object or experience by highlighting certain properties, downplaying others, and hiding still others. Each of the dimensions gives the properties that are highlighted.' (p. 163, emphasis added.)

The figure-ground principle plays a crucial role in focusing aware-ness on any group of stimuli, regardless of which sense you use. Whatever the figure, it determines the available information for the person to work with in shaping his perception. *This principle cannot receive over-emphasis.*

This immediately limits possibilities by setting a frame around a few certain pieces of information. Putting this principle with the one known as continuation, beliefs and perceptions perpetuate ad-infinitum. This equates to a habitual thought-emotion-behavior pattern–stretching out endlessly over time unless some element intervenes. Also, this figure-ground principle equates to the most basic category of data, nominal. Stimuli get divided into either figure or ground.

Several elements can alter the figure-ground relationship. Hypnotic language represents one of these elements. Removing the previous figure-ground perception lets the observer consider any part of the stimuli as they each hold equal standing. The former relationship between parts observed ceases. This permits voluntary figure-ground relationships so the observer can choose what parts he or she wants as the center of his attention.

How does it feel to you when you think about the amount of a project completed compared to focusing on the amount not completed? Stating that you have already completed 20 percent of an important project feels better than stating that you still have 80 percent to go. Conversely stating that you only have 20 percent left to complete feels better than stating that you have only completed 80 percent of the project. You can provide motivation by emphasizing one portion of the whole to serve as figure and the other as ground.

How does this principle of figure-ground apply to auditory stimuli? No doubt you have heard a wide variety of expressions over your lifetime. Some auditory stimuli may have been labeled as criticism, while other things you heard got labeled as praise or supportive. Which do you place as figure and which constitutes ground? If a person focuses on the perceived criticism in her life, a low sense of self-esteem or worth may result. But if a person focuses on the support and praise, leaving the criticism as blurred ground, then the result can be higher self-esteem.

Whatever you pay attention to, you always find more.

Whatever you pay attention to, you always find more. Countless stimuli bombard us through all of our senses. The ones we select to form the figure influence our beliefs about reality, including our self-image. Those stimuli that exist, but we ignored become ground and lose power to influence us. So, within the NLP model of stacking anchors and then collapsing them, we just lead the person to reverse figure and ground.

By switching the contents of figure and ground for a person with a low sense of self-esteem, evidence that supports personal worth comes to light. Within the individual's psyche, you may think of the conscious mind or primary awareness about self and the environment, as figure.

Secondary awareness, or unconscious mind, makes up the vast collection of stimuli known as ground. In the broadest sense, when you organize stimuli you perceive its results in some Gestalt. The label given this generally consistent collection of stimuli becomes the evidence supporting your beliefs and your beliefs become your reality. So any effective therapy amounts to what might be called *gestalt busting*, or at least Gestalt removal and replacement. The replacement Gestalt, or belief, gets chosen because it serves a need and purpose better.

Figure and ground also exists in our kinesthetic sense. One of the perceptual features that permit the fullest pain experience involves making the painful area the figure while the pain-free area constitutes the ground. You will find the language pattern, 'Play the Percentages', in the section dealing with perception. There I will give you an example that effectively reverses the figure-ground arrangement in the pain experience. This process significantly reduces the experience of pain by shifting awareness away from the area in pain to the area experiencing total comfort.

One of the perceptual features that permit the fullest pain experience involves making the painful area the figure while the pain-free area constitutes the ground.

This process significantly reduces the experience of pain by shifting awareness away from the area in pain to the area experiencing total comfort.

Likeness or Similarity

Grouping like kinds of stimuli together makes up the second perceptual feature. Gestalt psychology labels this organizing process as grouping for likeness or similarity. This grouping allows us to keep up with more information. We sort stimuli and form general categories that include more detailed or specific information within these categories. Recognize that the figure-ground arrangement plays a general role in this process of grouping for similarity. The stimuli that you decide are related combine to make the figure while the unlike kind makes up the ground. The general category of related stimuli determines the contents included.

The concept of similarity involving auditory information is essentially the same as the Milton model hypnotic language technique of phonological ambiguity. Earlier we included three uses of one homonym, sense, scents and cents. Once your mind hears one form of the word sense, you brain goes off on a hunt to determine which one of these possibilities fits the specific context. Whichever one seems to fit the context wins.

This also involves the Gestalt concept of simplicity that will be explained later. Suffice to state for now, that simplicity means we tend to first interpret stimuli in what we believe is the most simplistic form. This is the form that permits keeping our current perception intact by calling for the least complicated interpretations.

We tend to first interpret stimuli in what we believe is the most simplistic form. This is the form that permits keeping our current perception intact by calling for the least complicated interpretations.

Returning to similarity, I will cite an example of how these principles apply in hypnotic language. This case will provide an example of logic as a form of hypnotic language.

A client came in for counseling about a variety of issues. Among these was a conflict with her mother. This client was about 45 years old and her mother was around 70. This client's mother had a passive-aggressive style of relating to her daughter. The mother often attempted to emotionally manipulate her daughter into behaving the way the mother wanted her to. If the daughter did not comply with mom's wishes, mom in turn sought to make her daughter feel guilty for non-compliance. The daughter experienced an avoidance–avoidance conflict. Either the daughter complied with mom's request, though she did not really want to, or she would receive the mother's label of being an uncaring daughter.

The client and I talked about other interpretations that could also apply to the situation by accessing her secondary awareness and disassembling the gestalt (avoidance–avoidance–guilt, etc.) forced on her by her mother. Placing emphasis on alternative interpretations with caring about mother as the foundation, we examined other ways that the daughter could respond to her mother maintaining her desire to display care for her mother. I also cited counter examples of how a person may comply yet not really care and how a person may not comply yet truly care. I pointed out how compliance in the relationship with her mother centered around guilt so that the relationship rests on guilt and not, in fact, caring (illogical). And did she not find this actually contrary to her own purpose for relating with her mother? She strongly agreed.

Logic as a hypnotic language pattern came into play here and then drew upon simplicity placing the state of caring as the new and clear simpler interpretation of her own behavior. Then the client's gestalt, or belief system, became the source of her responses rather than the former avoidance–avoidance–guilt gestalt she had from her mother. Thus the client was able to offer the new gestalt to her mother instead of the one originating out of guilt. This permitted the daughter's care for her mother to become a useful foundation for responding and permitted the client to really associate into her feelings of caring about mother.

The new gestalt centered on the state of care as the figure and the similarity principle came at the end of the intervention by responding to her mother out of her caring for her. I mentioned to her that she could use any of the alternative interpretations and responses to her mother that now come out of her deep caring for her mother and I stated, 'I feel sure you can do these new responses with relative ease'.

Some words or terms possess elastic properties. They stretch to cover more than one meaning. The previous process stretches the words 'relative ease' to invite ease of accomplishing the task and ease as a state for both the client and her mother. Follow-up with this client revealed that she felt comfortable with her new responses and experienced no guilt. Putting her new gestalt to the test, her mother continued responding in the old way at first but this gradually subsided which allowed their relationship to include new and more satisfying turns. Most importantly the client persisted in her chosen care-based style.

This innate process involving similarity provides a pivot point for change. As an analogy, in the past, train yards used what was known as a roundhouse which was a means of pivoting the train engine to face another direction. A roundhouse is a round building with a straight piece of track within it. Sections of track outside the roundhouse touch the outer edge of the roundhouse from four or five different directions.

Think of the roundhouse being like the hub of a wheel with spokes attaching to it. The track at the entrance to the structure touches but does not hook up to the track in the roundhouse. The engine goes into the roundhouse from one direction and then the roundhouse rotates so the engine can come out aiming in a different direction down a different section of track toward the new destination.

> **Homonyms permit the opportunity for inviting the receiver to shift direction in his thinking.**

Likewise, homonyms permit the opportunity for inviting the receiver to shift direction in his thinking. Also recognize that the brain tends to think in terms of puns anyway—multiple meanings for the same piece of information. You *hear* a dog's bark, but you *see* a tree's bark; one word, yet appealing to different senses. In hypnotic language you then launch into a therapeutic metaphor utilizing trees. This would involve the need for dissonance reduction (looking for harmony) since confusion would set in due to the double use of bark and the tree metaphor. And just how will the listener reduce his dissonance? You provide this with whatever ideas or resources you present next.

43

Dissonance seems to make a person cognitively receptive for an explanation, so the first, most plausible explanation the listener hears stands a good chance of being accepted as legitimate. Accordingly, great hypnotists from Milton Erickson to Richard Bandler have seemed to delight in boring people to tears and/or confusing them.

Dissonance seems to make a person cognitively receptive for an explanation, so the first, most plausible explanation the listener hears stands a good chance of being accepted as legitimate.

The human mind seems to naturally think in puns due to this similarity perceptual principle. The following is an actual event illustrating how our mind naturally thinks in puns.

> While being served dinner at an Italian restaurant, the waiter offered the patron some freshly grated Parmesan cheese. Taking the offer, the diner watched the cheese shavings accumulate on her food and when she decided that she had enough, exclaimed, 'That's great' (grate).

You just can't help it can you? One category may store multiple meanings for flexible use. In hypnosis we find this very convenient. Knowing the process style of the brain enables the communicator to utilize this dynamic in more effective ways, increasing the likelihood of reaching the desired outcome. The Milton model pattern of phonological ambiguity utilizes this principle.

As noted earlier, humans tend to group perceived items into categories. The brain stores them this way as well. This principle can also come into play in another way. When you meet someone new who reminds you of someone else you already know, how easy is it to call the new person by the other person's name? This stems from the new person being similar in some significant way to the already stored information. The NLP concept of anchoring utilizes this principle.

From research of human memory, two applicable principles come into play with the similarity principle. These are *retroactive interference* and *proactive interference*.

Proactive interference occurs when old learning or memories interfere with learning new information such as calling a new friend by an old friend's name. This also parallels the general principle of conditioning where past learning gets triggered by familiar cues and gets applied to new, yet similar, conditions (a form of generalizing). New habits are difficult to develop in the place of old ones. This principle, whether it's called proactive interference or conditioning, perpetuates the incumbent style of functioning. Knowing the difference between past and present and remembering choice makes the crucial influence. Hypnotic language can assist in providing an effective stopgap between the old and new learnings by drawing on the unconscious mind to replace the old with the new.

Hypnotic language can assist in providing an effective stopgap between the old and new learnings by drawing on the unconscious mind to replace the old with the new.

Earlier I identified a concept referred to as *retroactive interference*. This process refers to new learning that interferes with recalling old learning. This means the way of shifting from ineffective choices to effective choices through new awareness shutting off the old. A simple example of retroactive and proactive interference involves travelling from the United States to Great Britain and then back to the United States. Originally, you learn to drive on the right side of the road in the U.S.A. and then find it difficult to remember you must now drive on the left side while in Britain. This represents proactive interference. The retroactive interference comes into play when you return to the U.S.A. and find it difficult to remove the new, left side driving style that you recently learned.

In the realm of psychotherapy and hypnotic language, one can draw upon retroactive interference to sustain change. When a person makes profound change she often finds it difficult to remember how she formerly thought, felt or behaved. All she can remember now pertains to her new style. This especially holds true when a person deeply associates into her new state or mindset. You can remind a person, through hypnotic language, to find and keep a future orientation thus invoking retroactive interference. Neuro-Linguistic Programming refers to this as Future Pacing. The client envisions applying her new learning and awareness in the future with great detail.

This principle of grouping similar items together allows shaping hypnotic language so it defies pre-existing categories.

This principle of grouping similar items together allows shaping hypnotic language so it defies pre-existing categories. This careful word arranging then forces the listener to abandon nominal data organizing. Similar information gets categorized together during perception and storage. But we tend to notice and react to stimuli that stands out from the norm (Hearst, 1977). When a stimulus presents itself as *unique* it forces *unique* processing and allows for special attending to the information the sender gives the receiver.

Notice that your reaction to the first use of the italicized *unique* is heightened compared to the second *unique*. To make an impression with someone, you must invite the receiver to experience novel stimuli and generate energy-filled neurological reactions. The shape and dynamics of hypnotic language cause this desired reaction in the receiver. It defies traditional processing and cannot just get placed with the old familiar data categories.

Because hypnotic language breaks grammatical rules and traditional communication standards, it sets up an irresistible response on the part of the listener.

Because hypnotic language breaks grammatical rules and traditional communication standards, it sets up an irresistible response on the part of the listener. The receiver must put the hypnotic language in the spotlight, excluding all other stimuli. This then induces trance.

Closure

Drawing from Gestalt psychology once again, another principle, known as closure, assists hypnotic language's effectiveness. Humans tend to fill in missing pieces in their perceptions. Each of us seems driven by the need to form wholes. *We fill in holes to have wholes*. Three, plus three equals… How quickly do you say 'six' in your head?

So you can trust that when you communicate with language in any form, and hypnotic language in particular, that the listener will ___ in the whole. How natural—doing otherwise causes discomfort and this drives us to complete the circle. Have you ever been speaking to someone and paused to find just the right word to express your idea? The listener often breaks the silence because they felt a need for closure. In our quest for closure we have all probably played the role of the silence breaker as well. The Milton model hypnotic language patterns of improper pauses and incomplete sentences utilize this principle.

> **You can lead a horse to water and be sure it'll know what to do next.**

You probably recognize that closure represents a relative to dissonance reduction. Leaving stimuli in incomplete form leads to dissonance so closure reduces the dissonance. And maybe now you're looking especially for the missing pieces you will fill in. How trance-like this becomes. But you can trust that your unconscious mind automatically looks out for your best interest and will continue doing so without your conscious effort. The use of this principle permits you to sometimes omit from your words the very _____ that you want the listener to most notice. You can lead a horse to water and be sure it'll know what to do next.

Simplicity

The concept of simplicity seems harmless enough, but this principle plays a significant role in both dysfunction and resolutions. Simplicity suggests that a person sensing a stimulus will draw upon the simplest explanation or perception for the stimulus or collection of stimuli. The perceiver will utilize the least amount of cognitive effort necessary to arrive at an explanation for the event or stimulus. The perceiver does not perceive beyond or below the surface of the circumstance and essentially jumps to conclusions about the meaning. During simplicity the perceiver reduces the data to the nominal or ordinal level of complexity.

Simplicity suggests that a person sensing a stimulus will draw upon the simplest explanation or perception for the stimulus or collection of stimuli.

When we 'fight' to sustain our existing beliefs about ourselves, others or life we manifest our drive for simplicity. Rather than suspending our beliefs and freshly assessing the specific new information as they relate to the whole, we tend to 'keep what we have' for that is much easier and simpler. The repercussions of not 'keeping it simple' involve our adjusting the meaning of the whole because of this new information. We don't like to do that because it is usually too much work.

While the interpretation may seem the most simplistic to the inter-preter, sometimes the meaning may actually be unduly complex and problematic. In part, simplicity means we tend to interpret in accordance with pre-existing beliefs. A person of low self-esteem may pass off a compliment as a fluke or dismiss it for some reason. If she accepts the compliment then she would be forced to re-examine her self-image. This might be too unsettling to her general mental organization so she chooses the more simple expla-nation of a fluke and just keeps her low self-esteem. In this case, the previous beliefs, however limiting they may be, function at a Meta-level to any desire for personal change.

As a meta-level phenomenon, these limiting beliefs forbid the acceptance of new information. Hypnosis 'bypasses' this phe-nomenon by introducing the client to even higher meta-levels that will give them permission to consider new and healthier alterna-tive frames of mind.

On numerous occasions, I (BB) utilize hypnotic language patterns in directing my client's attention to higher meta-levels within his unconscious mind. Spiritual Meta-identity levels provide excellent resources to 'bypass' limiting beliefs as the client's spiritual beliefs function Meta to his desire for simplicity. Also, in appealing to his higher spiritual beliefs, he feels much 'safer' in going there.

In some sense the desire for simplicity ties in with Piaget's concept of centering (1965). The perceiver does not look outside of his tunnel vision and so cannot consider multiple factors or explanations for what he perceives. This process of tunnel vision then naturally results in the perceiver displaying the concept of simplicity. However, this simplicity also operates as a function of the perceiver's cognitive, ego or moral developmental level. In a general sense, the higher the developmental level (a meta-level) of functioning that an individual occupies, the broader the awareness and the more a person can extend beyond self.

> **The highest levels of development yield a sort of fluid relationship between the conscious and unconscious so the person more easily accesses his unconscious mind.**

At higher developmental levels of functioning the perceiver possesses awareness that multiplicity of cause exists (Loevinger, 1976). The highest levels of development yield a sort of fluid relationship between the conscious and unconscious so the person more easily accesses her unconscious mind. This reduces the likelihood of perceiving with simplicity. By going Meta to these meta-levels, an individual can see each part that makes up the whole. From that position (dissociated to a higher witnessing position), the individual can 'choose' what beliefs best serve her interest in relation to the 'whole' that she desires for herself. And, because higher levels modulate lower levels, this meta position allows the client to discard limiting beliefs and to embrace beliefs that support 'wholeness'.

Hypnotic language then reduces or overrides simplicity since hypnotic language transports the listener from their conscious mind to their unconscious mind (the place of meta-level resources).

Hypnotic language also raises the listener's developmental level as they shift into operating from their unconscious mind. Each of the gestalt principles becomes malleable or arranged by choice when accessing the unconscious mind. Whether simplicity, closure, figure-ground, continuation or similarity, the unconscious mind permits the person to override their previous gestalt.

The other principle mentioned, aside from the unconscious mind, relates to human development levels. As noted in the last paragraphs, the person rises to higher levels of cognitive, ego or moral development when accessing and operating from the unconscious mind. This happens through many sources and hypnotic language represents one. Broader awareness and increased resourcefulness represent elevated developmental levels. Hypnotic language allows the person to developmentally ascend and then utilize their more sophisticated capacities within their unconscious mind.

In the unconscious mind, the whole notion of simplicity becomes mute. Operating from the unconscious mind severs the simplicity connection between the person and the stimulus. The unconscious mind functions Meta to any 'outside' stimulus as it can choose whatever interpretation of that stimuli it desires and which one(s) best serves its outcome. The stimulus then becomes open to interpretation. From this perspective, the perceiver then becomes amenable to a more accurate and useful simple explanation that they will be all too happy to embrace and thus apply to their life. So often the 'simplest' explanation that the client comes up with about any stimulus or event actually results from the most complicated and convoluted process which is anything but simple. In a moment I will give an example of what I mean by this.

However, simplicity combined with continuation often results in a person feeling reluctant to give up their 'simple' explanation in the name of security. Their life contains a sort of painful, yet predictable, routine.

The concept of simplicity plays a vital and powerful role in a client's hesitating to make change because the client feels they must shift to a more cognitively complex position. But once in trance the client then experiences cognitive flexibility (from meta-levels) and finds shifting perceptions much simpler. This affords the opportunity for the therapist to assist the client in finding a more effective interpretation or perception of events.

> The care of one of my clients, a 60-year-old married woman, serves as an example of simplicity and the use of hypnotic language to affect perception. She reported that she had suffered constant verbal and emotional abuse from her husband during her 43-year marriage. But since no tangible abuse occurred she felt unjustified in leaving her husband.
>
> Presently, he was drinking alcohol quite heavily. She told me that if her husband physically hit her or engaged in an affair she would immediately leave the marriage and not feel any guilt. She made it clear that her husband felt no desire to change his ways or the relationship in any way. She stated that the idea of leaving the marriage due to emotional and verbal abuse made her feel like a traitor. This not permitting herself to leave the marriage occurred in spite of past visits to an attorney and filling out various preliminary papers for divorce proceedings. She also went so far as to determine where she would live after the divorce and what activities she would use to fill in her life. But her traitor feelings prevented her from following through with her plans.

The simplicity principle displays itself by her choosing a rather traditional, socially prescribed perspective about her marriage and her role in it as a female. This global perspective (a meta-level for her) excluded any specific events, like abuse, in her marriage. This perception displayed the simplest form and placed her in a passive role to her husband. The role she perceived herself in as wife came from an external source (society) and required no independent thinking on her part.

Her dissatisfaction grew because some part of her knew that she was experiencing great harm by remaining in this marital arrangement. The dissatisfaction revealed dissonance, as two opposing belief systems came into conflict—societal expectations versus the part of her that knew of the intense suffering she experienced by remaining in this abusive relationship. The client expressed awareness of two general directions that would resolve the dissonance, leave and wrestle with feeling like a traitor or stay and learn to suppress her desires for personal freedom. Neither of these directions provided satisfaction because each had its drawbacks.

I first pointed out to her that if leaving the marriage felt like being a traitor then leaving must also display loyalty to something else. I asked her, 'If leaving the marriage led you to a traitor status, just what principle would you be loyal to by making this same choice?' This diverted her attention away from her husband and the constrictive beliefs to a sort of void, or yet to be identified set of powerful counter beliefs.

To address the limiting effect of her simplistic perception, I called on her already identified deep spiritual beliefs. Stepping into the spiritual realm (a meta-level of awareness) immediately removed her from society's prescription for her role in the marriage. This severed the simplicity ties. From here I asked if she held the belief that God resided in each of us. She affirmed this as her belief. I then noted how her husband actually treated God as he treated her since God resided within her. She was following the logic, which represented a form of hypnotic language. At this point I then noted that as long as she exposed herself to her husband's abuse, she conspired with her husband to treat God in a most highly disrespectful manner. She actually conspired with her husband to disrespect God.

This brought a flood of new awareness and an elevated perspective. While elevated and broader in awareness, the perspective actually consisted of very simplistic perceptions that held great truth for this client. She also came to quickly realize that she had accidentally placed her husband above God by obeying her husband rather than following the gentle, loving guidance of God, as she perceived it. This out-of-order hierarchy actually laid the groundwork for her distress, not the marriage or her husband, rather her simplistic perception. Once she yielded to her spiritual values and aligned her simplistic thinking with her meta-level values, she felt a peace and clarity about herself and her situation.

Dissonance Reduction

These Gestalt psychology principles of perception base themselves on what we believe to be the most powerful pre-existing principle. As mentioned earlier, each of us seems unavoidably compelled to make meaning of what we sense. Given this drive, if you communicate something unconventional to someone, the receiver must oblige human nature and attempt to process your message in order to understand it. This presents a major advantage and a huge, always open door through which to enter the unconscious mind. The unconventional portion of a hypnotic language pattern must fold itself within an otherwise traditional message. The unconventional portion of the message creates what Gestalt psychology refers to as dissonance.

Ericksonian hypnosis refers to this odd portion of a message as throwing the listener into confusion (Gilligan, 1987). Any time you cite counter examples you invoke dissonance in the listener. You can also lead the listener to a state of dissonance when you speak in a manner that includes information or words that defy the usual perceptual categories for information, hypnotic language.

Not only do we feel compelled to understand stimuli we sense, but Gestalt psychology suggests that our nature drives us to reduce dissonance. When a piece of a message is inconsistent with the whole or just doesn't seem to make sense, then confusion or dissonance sets it. Dissonance also occurs when two beliefs exist about the same event or when behaviors differ from beliefs. Because the listener is bound by the need to understand incoming stimuli and shave off inconsistencies, or reduce dissonance, the automatic next step involves the listener accessing and searching her unconscious mind in an attempt to make sense of the initially confusing message.

You might think of the listeners' need to understand your message as a sort of innate empathy. Now you and he gain entry into the resource-rich field of the unconscious mind. Once in the secondary awareness you can assist the listener in finding and associating into more resourceful ways. So the Gestalt concept of seeking dissonance reduction plays an important role in allowing effective hypnotic language. When using hypnotic language, you can rely on the dissonance reduction drive to stir a reaction in the listener of 'Huh, what in the world is this meaning?' The natural next step leads to the unconscious mind where the answer lies.

When a person experiences a feeling of being at odds with themselves, cognitive dissonance exists. Maybe all clients who come in for therapy find themselves in the midst of cognitive dissonance. Otherwise they feel, think and behave consistently—an absence of dissonance. Knowing the driving forces that play a role in and determine the expressed dissonance represents the crucial point.

◆　　In what way does the person experience a split?

◆　　What forces at deeper or higher levels seem at odds and create the dissonance?

Going into the unconscious mind permits reconciling these apparent adversaries. In an odd way you can use hypnotic language to create dissonance, then enter the unconscious mind to resolve the more crucial dissonance that brings the person in for therapy. The ambiguity language patterns in the Milton model create dissonance and open up the client for dissonance reduction.

> I will briefly present a case as an example of cognitive dissonance within a client and using cognitive dissonance in hypnotic language. This involves a woman who sought therapy for her depression. She had experienced a lot of trauma during her life. When she was 12 years old she saw her mother take her own life.
>
> The client had experienced a variety of other losses and disappointments throughout her life. In spite of these trials the client managed to finish college, get married and have a daughter. This woman brought in symptoms of anxiety and depression. She exhibited significant pessimism about almost any important part of her life. The pessimism served as a coping strategy for preventing loss and disappointment. But this strategy actually brought on the feelings of anxiety and depression. Additionally the client lived in the past (past orientation Meta-program). By focusing on her past, she generated this need for a coping strategy.
>
> The dissonance involved time, superimposing the past over the present and then generating emotions of anxiety and depression. But with nothing to support these emotions in the present, a discrepancy or inconsistency resulted. Her goal for therapy was to find relief from her anxiety and depression

while being able to enjoy her current life. She also felt confused and quite angry toward herself for knowing the dissonance existed yet not finding a resolution. She stated that she should be happy because of the life she presently had but she still felt depressed and anxious.

Several interventions took place to address her issues over the six therapy sessions. One particular intervention involved a simple one-line sentence that fits into the category of hypnotic language because it induced a trance. The sentence also utilized cognitive dissonance within it to assist resolving the cognitive dissonance within the client. Once we determined she did, indeed, use pessimism as a coping style I asked her, 'How will feeling bad keep you from feeling bad?'

(This sentence just identifies the away-from strategy and applies it to the state the person attempts to prevent. For the relationship avoiding person you could say, how will staying away from relationships keep you from ending up alone? This pattern demonstrates the NLP *sleight of mouth pattern applied to self.* See Hall and Bodenhamer, 1997b)

After a pause, and then some protesting to me that she doesn't do this process of pessimism to prevent pain and then another pause, the client clearly shifted.

The first pause likely involved internal processing at a lower level of cognitive awareness resulting in the protest. But a mismatch between beliefs and behavior was undeniable so she went back into her mind more deeply to make sense of this confusion-dissonance. I believe this accessed her unconscious mind. From this point forward the client quickly extinguished her pessimism and replaced it with perceptions that were consistent with her desired outcome. This new strategy generated the ability to enjoy the present rather than looking for how it may go wrong. Soon she stopped feeling the anxiety and depression. She reported experiencing an interesting state that she discovered after leaving pessimism, 'joy with a kick'. For her, this meant that she felt joy but that it possessed an added dimension of an energizing effect.

Continuation

The last component of Gestalt psychology that plays a role in hyp-notic language involves the concept of continuation. While this and the other gestalt principles primarily originated with visual perception, continuation also plays a role in thoughts, emotional states and behaviors.

Continuation refers to a person's habitual tendency to group stimuli in a way that minimizes disruptions.

Continuation refers to a person's habitual tendency to group stim-uli in a way that minimizes disruptions. Continuation involves simplifying a process to a single perception rather than two or more figures interacting. Any contrary stimuli get filtered out. When a person holds a belief, any belief, this belief becomes self-perpetuating and self-fulfilling. Two differing beliefs will not exist at the same time for very long. The dissonance reduction drive makes sure this doesn't happen. The one belief continues actively asserting and influencing thoughts, emotions and behaviors.

Any belief in place also determines what a person perceives. So the concept of continuation is played out by a person's continuing pat-terns of beliefs. This basic psychological element then influences perceptions, beliefs, states, thoughts or behaviors already in place. The influencing belief continues unless the person purposely chooses another belief. But then this new belief carries and dis-plays the same properties of continuation.

Continuation applied to beliefs, states, styles or strategies exhibits one of Newton's laws of physics. A body at rest-motion tends to stay at rest-motion. How does this fit within hypnotic language? Knowing the principle exists and comes as sort of factory equip-ment with each belief or state allows working with this principle. You can harness the continuation principle and allow it to work for you. By accessing the secondary awareness after dissociating from primary awareness, you can then assist the listener in choosing new, more useful beliefs or states. These new resourceful pieces will naturally perpetuate—just get the ball rolling and continue.

The process compares to simply shifting gears in a car or bicycle. Once in motion, you can shift gears and know that the moving object will simply continue its motion and apply this motion within the properties of the new gear, or belief, in the case of humans. Knowing this new belief or state will just naturally perpetuate, you can simply shift and then aim the new belief or state toward the circumstance that needs alteration.

Continuation is similar to the principle of generalizing. The client uses the same belief or state or strategy for any situation bearing the remotest resemblance to the point of origin. Even though the original context that constructed the belief no longer exists, the belief does not know that and it just keeps on working.

One of the most common reasons a person comes for therapy is to stop a runaway continuation. Continuation is similar to the principle of generalizing. The client uses the same belief or state or strategy for any situation bearing the remotest resemblance to the point of origin. Even though the original context that constructed the belief no longer exists, the belief doesn't know that and it just keeps on working.

Specific shifting to more resourceful beliefs-states-figures helps the specific situation. But installing the ability to identify cues for when and how to stop continuing one style and shift to another makes the person self-sufficient. Many of the hypnotic language patterns in the text utilize specific and general discontinuing approaches. This helps the listener stop a self-limiting style, replace it with a more effective one and continue with the new belief system.

The unconscious mind knows what to do with the information it gets. You may wonder if your message will get through to the person's unconscious mind in the way you intend. One of the traits of hypnotic language is purposeful vagueness. General messages with various principles or dynamics get sent out to the listener. The vagueness permits the receiver to take the general message and fashion it to fit her own needs.

Trust that the listener knows exactly what she needs. Give a person seven particular letters from the alphabet and let her spell a word using any or all the letters. She will make the word reflecting her individuality. Her unconscious mind is just right. If you sold shoes in a store and a barefoot person walked in, would you worry about what she will do? Trust the person will leave with what she came for, it is only fitting.

In general, hypnotic language reduces specific details in the external world into a select few categories of generalities for the listener. The listener ingests these generalities, first in a dissociated form, and then converts them back into specifics, as needed within the receiver.

Next, the listener associates into the details, albeit of a different nature, state or belief. So the order of events proceeds from the listener in an associated state about specific external information to dissociated forms of vague generalities. The receiver then converts the information back into associated state forms of specific internal information, albeit in different content forms.

Imagine an hourglass turned on its side. The left side consists of a large amount of details about external information in the environment. The right side consists of internal information in a similarly large amount of detail. In the middle exists a narrow passageway. Information about the environment must be converted into general pieces of luggage capable of holding vast amounts of information.

The most feasible way of transporting the external to the internal through the narrow space requires placing it in a less detailed form. The large amount of information gets reduced down to just a few pieces of large capacity luggage for the journey. By large capacity luggage, I mean using very general words like 'that', 'this' and 'it', because their flexible, vague references can represent many specifics, and be converted into a variety of meanings known best and only by the listener. The listener converts the large capacity general words into specific meaning within her own mind. It's sort of like taking dehydrated foods on a space flight. You can conserve room this way, ultimately taking more sustenance, and then just re-hydrating the food for consumption when you feel ready. And of course you can choose what you most want and the sender of hypnotic language always trusts that you know.

The hypnotic language patterns contained in this book possess considerable flexibility. You may remember and recite them or you may just read from a sheet once the person accesses the dynamics of her problem and associated states. At times we have handed a typed language pattern to a client and asked her to read it to herself. This proved effective for certain clients. The patterns may be used whole, in part or may simply provide launching pads for your own creations.

Each language pattern exemplifies some Gestalt psychology perceptual principles. Some focus on one or two, while others address several principles. And each pattern relies on the cognitive styles prevalent during childhood. The hypnotic language patterns are organized into five categories. These five include patterns addressing beliefs, time orientation, perceptual style (Meta-programs), spiritual issues and states of mind-emotion. You can recognize each pattern as they receive formal titles. The italic print before, during or after patterns acts as an explanation about the logic and purpose of the structure.

Manipulation?

It seems ethically important to address the possible concern on the part of the therapist that he or she may engage in manipulating the listener. Therapy seeks to steer the client to a higher and more effective style of functioning. The difference may be that in traditional therapy, the therapist engages his conscious mind with the conscious mind of the client and thus believes a positive, willful conspiracy exists. Yet, if significant change happens the therapist must still reach the driving forces within the unconscious mind.

> **If you help a hungry person to the food buffet who cannot reach it otherwise, do you consider this manipulation?**

If you help a hungry person to the food buffet who cannot reach it otherwise, do you consider this manipulation? Because, first and foremost, the client states where they want to go and the therapist just acts as a travel agent. Rest assured that the unconscious mind does not assume a passive role in the therapeutic process, whether or not the conscious mind is engaged by the therapist's conscious mind. In fact with hypnotic language you can bypass the conscious mind's obstacle and appeal directly to the source of personal power to assist the client in reaching his stated goal.

The road to the 'unpaved' world of the unconscious mind through hypnotic language begins with the paved conscious mind of both speaker and listener achieving deep rapport. You can only get off road by first travelling on road. With traditional therapy or hypnotic language the goal remains the same—assisting the client in reaching new and more effective awareness. The client then becomes aware of his own free will to employ this awareness or some other awareness. You will not 'make' anyone do your will. The client only reaches the choice point of true personal freedom. This point is the place of truly good mental health.

Part Two

Case Examples Showing the Application and
Effect of Hypnotic Language Patterns

Chapter Four

Language Patterns Addressing Beliefs, Behavior and Possibilities

> **Altering beliefs usually results in a change in behavior because we behave in ways consistent with our beliefs.**

Beliefs play a significant role in determining what we choose to do in our lives and what we choose not to do. The language patterns in this section challenge the source or the foundation of beliefs, point out the realm of possibilities and suggest alternative beliefs or behaviors that will lead to different response patterns. Altering beliefs usually results in a change in behavior because we behave in ways consistent with our beliefs. A person who holds the belief that he can trust others will approach others comfortably. But a person who believes others cannot be trusted will likely experience some discomfort when approaching others or may avoid others all together.

Another effective method for altering beliefs and behavior is through accessing the awareness of possibilities. In this place the person's awareness extends to a point that allows awareness of other possible outcomes and beliefs. Resources exist outside the unwanted belief in a sort of storage form. These are yet to take form; all things are truly possible. Here, no beliefs are held, they all exist as available options like clothes hanging in your closet. The hypnotherapist guides the client to a dissociated position that operates Meta to the client's perceived problem state(s). Once outside the problem belief, the client realizes new possibilities.

Beliefs can also change by adopting different behaviors. New information can come to light through the new behavior. This in turn brings different results and different information becomes available to the actor. In essence, the person puts fear to the test. At this point a discrepancy may exist between prior beliefs and current information.

For example, an individual may behave passively because she fears that if she speaks her mind, others will reject her. This passive person generalizes this belief to all people. But one day, this passive person asserts herself, speaking her mind and voicing her opinion. To her surprise, the people who hear this opinion react very supportively. This new behavior brings a new result and these new results can lead to new beliefs about self, others and the world. The new experience leads to a new map.

The foundation of a belief can change from the inside out, choosing new beliefs and behaving accordingly, or it can change from the outside in, behaving differently to create new information and then change the foundation.

The *foundation of a belief* can change from the inside out, choosing new beliefs and behaving accordingly, or it can change from the outside in, behaving differently to create new information and then change the foundation. The difference between changing the foundation and behaving differently to change the foundation is the source of the change. Changing the foundation just involves the person choosing a different belief and behaving accordingly. The behavior source of belief change occurs when the person changes her behavior but initially keeps her old belief until the behavior consequences disprove the old belief. It happens when a person says, 'I don't believe this (the client's strategy) will work but I'll try it anyway.' Then it works so that she changes her belief about self, others and or life.

So you can address beliefs using any of these three paths: foundation of beliefs, the awareness of all possibilities and the ripple effect on beliefs brought on by different behavior. Any one of these paths offers leverage for the hypnotherapist to effectively alter thoughts, emotions and behavior. The hypnotic language patterns that follow exemplify these three principles for making change.

> **So you can address beliefs using any of these three paths: foundation of beliefs, the awareness of all possibilities and the ripple effect on beliefs brought on by different behavior.**

Round Table: Relationship Issues

This example strays from hypnotic language, per se. Although it does involve communication with the unconscious mind it incorporates behavior as the primary form of communication. This intervention draws from the idea that actions speak louder than words—nonverbal communication. The case involves a woman in her mid-40s.

The client brought many issues for discussion and change. These hinged on a long-standing disconnection from her 'truest self' that also limited her access to her unconscious mind. It seemed that most of her significant relationships were filled with various conflicts. Through the course of therapy the client developed more trust in her unconscious mind. She began resolving issues with her mother, her daughter and one of her sons. However, after dealing with her most pressing issues, she mentioned having conflict with her older son. While not as intense as the other conflicts, the disagreements between her and her older son still bothered the client.

This client described how she and her older son seemed to go through relationship cycles. For a while they would get along well but then one of them would start an argument. The dynamics of this relationship apparently called for each of them to take turns as to who would start the argument. The issues utilized for the conflict rarely amounted to anything really important. It just seemed essential that they argue and alternate who initiated the process. It seemed almost as though they got into these arguments as a substitute for expressing the positive feelings they each had for the other.

Using this information about her dynamics, I sent the client off on an assignment. I first asked if either she or her son had a round dining table in either of their homes. She stated that her son did own a round dining table in his home. I then asked that she comply totally with the instructions that I would give her and that no matter what she thought about the assignment she was to carry it out to the fullest. I instructed the client to ask her son for his fullest cooperation in this assignment and to tell him that she really needed him to help her with this project.

The assignment involved the client going over to her son's home and both of them going into the dining room where the round table sat. They were to stand across from each other at the dining table facing each other. Then they each faced opposite directions so that they could walk around the table in the same direction. It did not matter who started the procedure but one of them was to say 'go' and they were to walk slowly around the table keeping pace with the one in front. Whoever started the process kept walking at least one full rotation around the table until the other decided to say, 'switch'. At this point they turned around and walked the other direction led by the other person. This was to go on until the one now following decided to say, 'switch'. The direction reversed again and they continued alternating in this manner until she decided it was enough.

The purpose of the exercise was to communicate with her unconscious mind by accessing the relationship dynamics with her son and then promoting conscious control over them. The idea being that, after she repeated this repetitive process, she would just decide enough is enough and put a stop to it. These relationship dynamics are similar to the assigned process of the two of them alternating who follows whom around the table. Each alternates calling the action to start much in the way they argue. The deeper purpose was to replace their roundabout way of relating with a more direct and constructive style. The leading and following also encouraged a deeper connecting and awareness of the other one, promoting empathy.

When this client came back for her next session, I asked how the assignment went. She began getting tearful and through her tears she said that the process went fine. I asked her what she learned. She said that she learned her son really cared about her and that she felt very good about this. I had contact with this client some months later and she reported that her relationship with her son continued to go very well. She described a positive and mutually supportive relationship.

How Do You Know That You Know What You Know?
Questioning Beliefs' Foundation

> **The concept of comparisons plays an essential role in forming the beliefs, states of mind, thoughts, emotions and behaviors of every human.**
>
> **People cannot state a belief about themselves without possessing awareness of other perspectives.**

The contents within this language pattern represent one of the more influential concepts within hypnotic language and general psychic make-up. Each statement of opinion or judgment or general decree containing a label comes from an internal comparison. The internal comparison may start with noticing an external stimulus but comparison and meaning occur internally.

As one of my (BB) students said, 'All meaning is an inside job'. Nothing in itself has meaning until a 'meaning making machine' called a human brain comes up to it and gives it meaning. The only way an element can remain without a label or value is by existing in a vacuum. There, no comparisons exist. In real world existence, elements take on meaning from comparisons to other elements. This means the same thing as the NLP presupposition that states, 'All meaning is context dependent'. Alfred Korzybski introduced this concept in his classic work *Science and Sanity* (1933/1994). This phenomenon allows for the possibility of reframing (changing meaning). When hypnotherapy works, it directs the client in 'reframing' unwanted beliefs and concepts.

People cannot state a belief about themselves without possessing awareness of other perspectives. Consider the person who states they lack social poise. To say this, the same person must contain awareness of what makes up social poise. Otherwise, the person could not state such a claim. The claim results from comparing his own behavior to what he perceives as social poise and making a statement about the gap between his behavior and some idea known within. The behavior occupies primary awareness while the known idea, and all other ideas, resides within secondary awareness.

> **The crux of therapy in general and hypnotic language in particular consists of drawing on the contents of secondary awareness and converting this to primary awareness.**

The crux of therapy in general and hypnotic language in particular consists of drawing on the contents of secondary awareness and converting this to primary awareness. The process of shifting from primary awareness to secondary awareness receives assistance from what amounts to linguistic loosening tools. This includes creating dissonance and time disorientation with spoken words.

Words with double meanings (phonological ambiguity) create dissonance because they create confusion in the listener. The person hearing the word with double meaning must decide which use of the word fits the context of the overall message. When a word does not fit the context of the rest of the message the mismatch is dissonance. To resolve the dissonance, the listener searches within himself or herself to examine meaning choices and decide which meaning to use. In the process, a trance happens. Some subtle use of double meanings appears with 'affix', 'worth labeling' and 'nothing to it'.

> **When a word does not fit the context of the rest of the message the mismatch is dissonance. To resolve the dissonance, the listener searches within himself or herself to examine meaning choices and decide which meaning to use. In the process, a trance happens.**

The hypnotic pattern below also uses perceptual filters, in particular figure-ground from Gestalt Psychology, to invite a shift of focus from what is not ideal to identifying and drawing upon the contents of what is ideal. The question of 'what are you not doing when labeling', points the person to her secondary awareness. This also pre-supposes that all resources exist within the individual. But you know this for we all carry within us adequate resources to attain our individual outcomes. Dissonance reduction needs are played up to in the first line. And the overall pattern involves the essential big four solution steps, associating into the problem-state, dissociating from the problem-state, associating into the resource-state and then applying it in life.

Just how is it that you know what you think you know... and before that? You must find some reference to which you pay deference. The only way you can state any claim about self is by first examining your current act. Once you determine it, this information must be compared to some source to observe the similarity or differences.

You affix a label to the gap between actual and desired outcome. But this label does not fix anything. The greater the gap the stronger and more condemning the label. And labeling only stalls the progress of moving toward your desired way. You end up living in empty space, there's nothing to that. What do you not do while you label? Now notice the location of this reference source within you. And you may say you use someone outside of yourself as the measuring stick but don't get stuck on the stick. What in you knows to use this outside example? Feel it resonate and identify itself. In order to choose an external you must first consult an internal, now isn't this so.... you can identify, feel and rely on using this internal knowing of what you want to be you are, now aren't you? Naturally, you know.

Instead of noticing and labeling the gap, trying to fill and close the gap with labels, consider how you know what you know, the substance, you know? Look very closely at the contents of the most desired outcome. What do you find makes this up, just looking, no obligation? This is worth labeling. What do you feel finding this?

Now you know you must contain the where with all within for performing as desired because you know you are not yet you will, won't you? You can only know this because you know that…you know what the desired performance is, don't you? Look, listen and feel the full contents of the most desired you hold within to the full infinite depth, no space, just feel the fullness. Now how will you use what you really know n-o-w, behaving consistently from this point? Where to begin keeping and using?

Note: I believe spelling out certain key words or concepts, promotes deeper processing of them by the listeners. By providing the raw material, the letters in order, you allow the listener to draw his own conclusion-awareness. This makes conclusion-awareness self-generated and more likely the listener will associate into the idea. This process represents the difference between dogma and experiential learning. Self-generated conclusions also avoid clients' bids for control that get labeled resistance. In a very general sense, spelling out words with the listener making the meaning from the letters equates to the overall process within hypnotic language; in this case, letters instead of words to be assembled by the listener.

A Stones Throw: Addressing Feelings of Frustration or Futility

The words here constitute a rather simple metaphor of a person's actions and the effects of those actions. Factors playing a role in the process include patience, the sphere of desired influence, the size of the effort by the person and the overall universal interconnection of all elements. In the language patterns I give water living traits, which appeals to the childhood sense of animism. The general theme in the story also promotes internal cooperation for the listener as the 'waves' all communicate, share and work together to reach a common goal. Describing the stone sinking through the water to the deepest point invites the listener into a deeper trance. This hypnotic pattern could easily fit in with the patterns affecting mental-emotional states but I feel that it also addresses beliefs about self, others and even the larger world.

Bodies of water, they take their cues from the surrounding land, the shore it's called. The body of water will adjust itself to the shape of the shore. Water also lives by certain principles. Among these is communication. Water actually communicates within itself through waves. One wave tells another wave that tells another wave to wave to the next one. Very cooperative, this water. Very inclusive in its communication as well. When making waves, all parts of the water get included in the circle of communication, ripples spreading out from the center in a circle.

Now some principles of water communication also exist. Two in particular include the size of the wave and the time from center to shore arrival. If a stone lands in the middle of the water you know what happens, the stone slowly sinks deeper and deeper finally coming to rest way below the surface. And news spreads fast to all parts. The size of the stone determines the size of the wave. And please realize as the size of the stone thrown increases so does the effort needed to place it in the center. Heavy objects need more umph! to move them. Yet these heavy objects reward with a bigger splash.

The other part of the water communication principle relates to the size of the body of water. The larger the body the longer it takes for waves to reach their final destination, maybe you could call it shoring. So please realize patience is needed if you throw a stone in a large pool, provided you want to have the waves reach the shore. The bigger the stone and the larger the body of water, the more effort and patience you need to remember beforehand. So how do you make waves? It's just a stone's throw away. And how appealing it is to hear and see the results spread to all parts, knowing the inevitable and feeling this now.

Clouds: Being Part of the Universe—Not Isolated From It

Do you believe we live in an 'interconnected' world? Many do. In this pattern my purpose relates to this universal sense of connectedness. Using clouds and their life cycle as a metaphor for humans, the words aim to provide some reassurance as to each person's inevitable intertwining with all other elements. Additionally, by suggesting that people exist both before and after a visible human form, this allows for a stronger sense of security. Within the description rests an underlying theme of our existence as a part of a larger scheme orchestrated by a Grand Being. This pattern assumes that we are not alone as individuals in the universe. This sense of being alone and or ending up alone is a common issue for clients. Aloneness drives a preventative strategy that encourages poor or hurried choices. In this pattern I seek to install within the client the belief that in fact we are never alone.

Sometimes when you do not see something you forget its presence. This seems partly because you put too much belief into your powers of perceiving. You always miss some parts when perceiving but you forget this when you believe your perceptions fully and accurately take in your surroundings. With this in mind think about moisture being in the air. Even when you can't see it or feel it, you know it's there. This is partly so because some people measure the moisture in the air with humidity and dew point readings. Looking up into a cloudless sky may give you the visual impression that no moisture exists there. You get reminders though when the process of condensation happens. This makes clouds appear out of thin air. The moisture makes itself known. Clouds make clear that change is in the air.

This condensation process makes for clouds. These puffy hues of gray that sometimes look like cauliflower, drift across the sky expanding as they go. It seems the bigger they get the darker hue they show. The darkest hues come just before the release of the moisture the cloud was holding. This makes the cloud vanish. The cloud resulted from an invisible process involving moisture, dust, air pressure and temperature. The visible cloud comes from the creative event. A cloud can not be if moisture is not. It is almost like being born. Where do we come from before we are conceived by moisture, dust and air; the trinity? Clouds go through life spans just like we do. They are born, evolve, accomplish certain goals and then revert to their previous invisible forms. Many different types of clouds come into existence. Certain traits bring identifying names like cyrus, stratus or cumulo-nimbus. Maybe you've heard of such terms. Some clouds rain, some snow, some hail and others blow over or decorate the otherwise indistinguishable uniform sky.

Clouds occupy certain altitudes. Some clouds hover low to the ground. We call these clouds fog. Other clouds slide by high above the ground as frozen white, semi-transparent sheets. Clouds are never wrong. They just are and are just right whether forming as a group or going solo. They never participate by precipitating before the perfect time. They always know when and how without doubt. Never self-centered, clouds are clear about purpose, always naturally fulfilling. They provide fine examples of faith and hope too. Is there ever just one drop of rain? And conscientious clouds are, they never let a single piece of moisture leave by itself and they always recycle. And clouds know how to feel really good too. By all means remember cloud nine.

Have a Ball: Beliefs about Competence

The words contained in this pattern appeal to a person's deeper 'knowingness'. These words presuppose that some part of the listener really knows exactly how to accomplish any goal. In NLP one of the key presuppositions states that each individual has the necessary resources to accomplish his purpose. The secondary awareness gets highlighted in this collection of words. The early section provides a path for the conscious mind to latch on to the details, as it is prone to do, and then proceeds to the unconscious mind.

The two teams in the story relate to the listener's moderate to low self-confidence. The story is used for directing the client to internal resources that can help improve his relationships. Calling on past success, a positive resource occurs by referring to the professional player's accomplishments that surely must precede his rise to the professional ranks. The players could not have risen to the ranks of professional were it not for previous successes. This remembering of what and where success occurred in the past is then moved forward into the present and future (a Meta-stating process). The general dynamics of losing and reclaiming self-confidence play within this pattern.

> Last night I watched a football game on television. One team wore their colored jerseys indicating they were most likely the home team while the other team wore white jerseys. Neither team had a good win–loss record so the game seemed evenly matched. Most of the players were fairly new to the professional ranks except two on one team. I set this up this

way to illustrate how beliefs influence outcomes. The team carries a belief about their ability to play effectively or not. Each individual on the team also carries a belief about his own competence. These may or may not be consistent.

What probably is true is that each of these players once carried very high beliefs about his own competence. No player could ever be on a professional team if he did not once demonstrate his ability to win. And we all know beliefs precede and are consistent with ability. Maybe when he played college ball or maybe when he played in high school. But no doubt he once felt certain of his competence, he believed he could and would win. He knew and remembered how to win. Well in this game last night both teams demonstrated their current beliefs that differ from their past beliefs, they believed they could not use their competence. They seemed to forget what they believed about their ability and how to use it. The game illustrated very well the old adage, use it or lose it. Both teams tried to lose it.

So I began to wonder if all the players, except two, forgot their beliefs about their high ability and where might it be stored. One player had not scored a touchdown all year and this game was the 12th, amnesia at its worst. Yet sometimes when you look inside yourself it becomes very difficult to do so objectively. So much seems at stake that you lose some perceptual ability, you know?

So where is the objective, unbiased storage of beliefs containing high ability? It suddenly dawned on me, the ball! After all, who scored more touchdowns and field goals than any player? The ball! Who was present during each tackle or run and catch for a touchdown? The ball, wow! It contains such a rich storehouse of memories about how to play well, score and win. Just ask the ball because it knows how to score and win. It has done so for many individual players and teams. Each scoring player carries something that knows how. Follow the ball and let it tell you how, guiding you to the score. To win you just need to have a ball.

Leaving Desires: Unexpressed Desires

We all experience desires of various kinds. Likewise, we can suppress them or we can express them. Suppressing desires leads to unhealthy tendencies in humans. How? Because the desire will likely gain expression but in some convoluted form or it will at least exert significantly undue influence on the holder. Yet, expressing desires in impulsive, raw, unbridled or disrespectful ways often violates human and spiritual laws.

The process dynamics of suppressing desires in humans resembles the function process of human laws. These laws do not address the root of the desire or the internal discrepancy giving rise to the desire. The law just suppresses the desire without exploring its deeper intention. The words making up this pattern attempt to address the deeper positive intention that moves a desire to conscious awareness. Once the root of the desire is made known a more effective way of expressing it can happen. Resolution can usually be effected.

This pattern also addresses the initial fear that often stops a person from tuning in and acting on his desires. The first step in the process of giving life to a desire often involves an exaggerated version of the actual need. It is like what happens after you sit for a long time. When you first get up you stretch and move a lot, then you settle back down. People often forget the first phase of expressing a long suppressed need is just this, the first phase and not the final outcome. The reference in the language pattern invites the listener to go above and beyond the surface desire finding his more substantial and useful drive.

The early part of the pattern sets the stage for helping the client in becoming more receptive to the concepts presented later in the pattern. The early part of the pattern also seeks to garner his participation within the process.

> Now you may need to shift if you want to get this and you know you ... can shift and get this like catching a fly ball. You go where it is if you want to get an out in the inning to get out of the inning. Sort of like laws are after the fact, closing the barn door after, instead of before, but more important is

knowing, what drove the animals to mooove out of the barn. Laws do not change the desire they only leave the desire pent up. Instead of finding out why, the door closes.

What laws do you live by without finding out why the law exists, leaving pent up desires? If you know, when you know, what will you know and what will the leaving desire leave you with after the initial stretch from being pent up allows full extension of the deep desire coming to light...your way. Now following the path lighted by your desire as it propels toward it's known destination, seeing and feeling its way, leaving ... desires ... freedom, but you know these now and always have and will use them now, won't you?

Without a Trace: Beliefs About Personal Strength

This hypnotic language pattern is essentially just a metaphor describing the challenge in the drive for personal independence. The story describes the emotions associated with the struggle for independence against an antagonist. We rely on egocentrism to work for we believe that the listener will associate into the story and apply it to himself or herself. The listener is also invited into the essential steps involved in the change process. This includes associating into the problem state, then shifting to associate into a resource state and applying this resource to the problem state. The story also addresses possible objections or obstacles often encountered along the way to reaching emotional and behavioral independence. Once the story has described the benefits of independence, the state within the listener becomes self-reinforcing and continuation takes over.

> This is the story of inkling, a baby pen. Inkling was born of two parents, the Fountains. Each parent was rather strict and provided many rules for inkling to live by. There were many activities inkling could not do and only a few that inkling was permitted to do, and these were not without parental supervision. In this case, supervision equaled control. Inkling was told how to move and what moves could be made. As inkling grew up and continued getting bigger, he [*choose corresponding gender throughout*] began wanting to make his own letters but his parents forbade this.

They required that he not only copy their letters, but to actually just trace over the letters they already made. He longed to create his own letters and not just trace over those already made by his parents. He knew no room existed for discussing the issue. He felt like he had no rights. His parents would simply not hear of his concerns. After all, this was the way his parents and their parents before learned to make letters. Of course inkling realized that no new letters were ever created because the same old ones were gone over and over without ever breaking out into different letters, how constrictive.

Inkling continued carefully complying with his parents' demands all the while plotting how to break free of the restrictive lines. He knew that inside him was a free flowing stream of letters including the entire alphabet. New letters and, more importantly, new combinations of letters leading to completely new words. How exciting, just to consider the possibilities. He managed to maintain an acceptable surface appearance to his parents. But he knew deep inside resided the ever-flowing realm of beautiful curves and lines. Inkling also knew his parents were trapped and could not rise above and stop their own confining circumstances. They felt compelled to always keep their tip to the paper. For them he felt compassion. But this would not inhibit his essential mission. In fact it made it more compelling.

Inkling recalled his experiences with others and the tales others told about seeing or making different letters and words. In fact inkling read these other letters but was not allowed to make them, let alone create new words forming new combinations. He knew if freedom was to happen he would have to take matters into his own hands. About this he was certain and this awareness itself provided a degree of comfort. The exit door was illuminated. Inkling also knew his parents would feel frightened by his altering and their reaction might look like anger. That or they may just laugh at him but this would only be to keep their fear at bay. This comforted him as well. He could decode their lines now and this resulted in immunity to their attempts to keep him in line.

Having imagined free-flow writing for quite some time, inkling realized that nothing short of truly experiencing this would do. Filled with awareness, certainty and exuberance, he suddenly clicked into action, emerging from the long imposed confinement. Tip touched paper and ignited a steady stream of letters and words long known. He felt exhilarated as actions aligned with purpose. How much easier writing became because he removed the restrictions and limitations to exhibiting that which was already in him. This now felt so natural, comfortable and free to inkling. He knew all that he knew is true.

The Elastic Band: Beliefs About Rigid Use of Strategies

Have you ever 'pushed' too far in the only direction you know to go in? Well, in this story we consider the consequences of over-using an effective behavior or response style. If a person uses only one strategy when trying to solve any problem, it will eventually backfire. Just because the strategy worked once or twice at crucial times it does not mean it will work every time. But sometimes people over-generalize and rely on one strategy that does not fit for all contexts. This over-generalizing can actually *be* the presenting problem when the client thinks the problem is that the situation won't yield to a tried and true solution. Eventual ineffectiveness results from over-reliance on any one strategy for dealing with self or the environment. It seems that fear underlies the motivation for applying a single strategy to all issues.

> **If a hammer is your only tool then you will treat every issue as if it is a nail.**

If a hammer is your only tool then you will treat every issue as if it is a nail. This familiar phrase reflects the inflexibility in one dimensional problem solving. The story in the following language pattern provides a strategy for preventing an undesired outcome and it reveals how a presupposed preventative strategy can backfire and lead to a dead end. The story accents various states driving the strategy. Noting states that result from the eventual limitations allows the listener to step into these states. This leads to the next step in the story, which is to consider the possibility of a new strategy but not acting on it yet. The purpose of identifying the urges not acted on is because most people, in their unconscious mind at least, already know what they want to do and how to do it. They just hesitate for various reasons.

Embedded in the later portion of the story is a suggestion that these new mentally rehearsed response styles eventually overtake the old and simply emerge as a result of frequent rehearsing. This emerging then brings more desired outcomes and more resourceful states. The perceptual styles of dissonance, continuation and similarity allow this story's effectiveness. The dynamics of this story use the mind's natural filing system of placing similar pieces of information together.

> **The dynamics of this story use the mind's natural filing system of placing similar pieces of information together.**

The effectiveness of the language pattern depends upon the client's matching your words in accordance to the words in his filing system. This makes use of the matching style of the mind's filing system. But the variance occurring later in the story, compared to the initial 'similar' contents previously stored in the categories of the mind, create a sort of thought virus contaminating the old information and its usual response style.

The same dynamic plays out when matching a person's emotional intensity and then leading them to a lower emotional state. Match and then lead with the hook you create by matching the client's words. Naturally comparing the new story with the old information forces awareness of and reduction of dissonance. By offering a more desirable outcome, planted within the new strategy mentioned, invites converting the old, one-dimensional style into the new, flexible style.

This is a story about a band that calls itself The Elastic Band. The name is ironic because they are anything but flexible. Not that they aren't popular, they are, but they only play one tune. No matter how they try, the band cannot seem to play a different melody. They begin to shift from the usual tune into a different one but always loop back into the familiar. They can stretch but always snap back. This one tune is exceptionally well liked by their fans and audience. The band is even amazed at their popularity. Everyone likes their tune so this is the only one they play. People drive in droves from miles around to hear the band play their one long song. Most of the time the elastic band does one or more encores. The band sort of fell in love with their own song too, but mostly because it brings them popularity.

This immense popularity leads the band to begin touring around the country playing their song to many more people who have yet to hear it. They meet with the same response, applause and waves of adoring fans. While this point is a great one to experience, the audience begins longing for something more from the band. The band members also begin longing to play something new. However, none of the band members dare play a different tune, lest they risk losing their popularity.

While continuing to play the same song in public, the individual members of the elastic band begin secretly experimenting individually. Without informing the other members, each practices playing different tunes in their own home. Each feels rather afraid, embarrassed and a little guilty. At the same time they feel compelled to let loose the varied tunes they can hear in their own heads. They can no longer keep these new tunes and harmonies pent up.

In the meantime, the elastic band continues playing their same single tune without variation. While a faithful core audience continues coming to see and hear the band play their tune, fewer and fewer people show up for shows. The band tries shortening their song, expanding their song, playing it slower, then faster but the listeners continue dwindling. All the while, each member keeps up secret practices of their new, and now expanding, repertoire. As a result of their private developments, each member feels a widening gap between what they play publicly and what each practices privately. Increasing feelings of discomfort continue, as the band members are each uncertain as to what is happening or where this is all leading.

In one of their many performances to the shrinking audiences, a very shocking turn of events occurs. Suddenly, and with no warning or planning, one of the members unconsciously breaks into a totally new tune, unheard in public before now, right in the midst of the band's playing their old familiar. First amazement and confusion by the other band members, this gives way to an odd anger at the mutineer, which then leads to knowing this is the way to go so they eagerly follow.

Feelings of excitement, joy and awareness of infinite new possibilities follow. You know how you can practice new ideas and ways just in your mind. And these ways depart dramatically from the usual repertoire. Continuing practice begins causing the awareness of new to become known more deeply and then sort of take over or commandeer the choice making system and devise, leading to unconscious and now automatic changes and variations from the former to easily and naturally displaying more and useful methods. Rather than reacting with surprise just leap ahead, allowing eagerness, joy and awareness of infinite possibilities to follow.

The Last Dance: *Beliefs About the Benefit of Procrastinating*

In this pattern we focus on the common problem behaviors of avoiding issues and putting off acting on them. In the presentation, I address the desired outcome for the client and then build up the intensity through anticipation, only to suddenly leave the client empty handed. First, the pattern induces a light trance through methods of similarity (chance). Next, I introduce awareness of the finiteness of human time (sort of like planting a 'time bomb') followed by the detailing of event transactions at the dance, which allows the person to drift along to the desired bump. The bump is designed to awaken the person into knowing that time is limited and encourages the person to take advantage of opportunities in the present.

The listener is then taken into the future and shown an undesired outcome produced by his avoidance strategy. Next, he is brought back into the present and sent on a mission seeking fulfillment and his desired outcomes. At the end of the pattern, I do not give a suggestion as to the application of the moral of the story. This plays upon his need for completion, as the listener will simply fill in the blank (a Future Pace) with his desired outcome. Additionally, dissonance reduction motivates the person in reconciling the difference between the client's desired outcome and the undesired outcome described in the story.

> This is one of those stories about time and chance. If you think too much about time and chance, chances are you will drift off into a trance. But do not worry, you will come out in

time. This series of events take place at a dance. And just what is not a dance of some kind in life? But this sort of dance is the kind with music playing in a particular time creating rhythm for dancing to. Two particular characters take part in this dance with time and chance.

These people already know each other and arrive at the dance separately. They decide to dance with others there but vow to save the last dance for each other. The evening progresses and they each dance a lot with many different people enjoying themselves thoroughly. But all the while they keep in the back of their mind the special significance of the last dance and who it will be danced with. Anticipation grows, as each knows the value of the irreplaceable ceremony. Bonding and feeling the emotional synergy like no other. While dancing with others they continue keeping an eye on the other, imagining the finale … . Band dismantles, lights out, going home empty handed.

You may say that the band will announce the upcoming last dance but what if they don't? And where else do last dances and chances occur without announcing and how will you know, before or after?

Rotation: Belief Change Process

The four parts for either sustaining or dismissing a belief are certainty, doubt, being unsure and disbelief (Hall & Bodenhamer, 1999). To undo a belief you start with certainty then produce doubt. Following doubt you produce a sense of being unsure and finally you end up with disbelief.

In the following pattern, I address the dynamics involved in belief formation. The four parts for either sustaining or dismissing a belief are certainty, doubt, being unsure and disbelief (Hall & Bodenhamer, 1999). To undo a belief you start with certainty then produce doubt. Following doubt you produce a sense of being unsure and finally end up with disbelief. At this point the belief disappears allowing a person to choose a replacement belief that will increase his chances of obtaining the desired outcome. The language pattern below describes the belief replacement process and uses the metaphor of changing a flat tire.

The start of the pattern process refers to time orientation. The pattern represents time metaphorically in the general process of tightening and loosening that we use regularly in the fastening of such devices as lids and lug nuts. The purpose of this is to loosen and tighten represented beliefs of the past and the future respectively. You can utilize these directions in taking a person back in time to before his current limiting belief and thus render it non-existent.

When you have a person conceptually before a limiting belief, you allow that person to create an empty place where he once had a limiting belief. If the person is conceptually 'before' he installed the limiting belief, the limiting belief doesn't exist there. This will give him permission to install a more resourceful belief from this Meta position.

The same four steps of certainty, doubt, being unsure and disbelief that allow a belief to influence us now apply again but to the constructing of a resourceful belief. In constructing a resourceful belief, follow these steps: 1) move from disbelief to unsure; 2) from being unsure to doubt; 3) from doubt to certainty; and 4) then you tighten the new belief in place. You can present this pattern in general before or after belief intervention or apply it to a specific belief elicited from the client. If the latter applies, you will simply name the specific belief removed and the replacement belief at the appropriate times within the pattern. This pattern works as a linguistic Time-Lining process. Note the use of temporal and spatial presuppositions in this pattern with the use of words like: past, future, forward, right, left, behind, front, preceded and forward.

When you have a person conceptually before a limiting belief, you allow that person to create an empty place where she once had a limiting belief. If the person is conceptually 'before' she installed the limiting belief, the limiting belief doesn't exist there. This will give her permission to install a more resourceful belief from this Meta position.

> **In constructing a resourceful belief, follow these steps:
> 1) move from disbelief to being unsure; 2) from being
> unsure to doubt; 3) from doubt to certainty; and 4)
> then you tighten the new belief in place.**

Have you ever noticed how we arrange the rotation of items such as lids or other types of fastening devices? Notice how tightening involves turning the lid to the right and loosening involves turning to the left, how curious. Now be aware that most people's minds organize time from left to right representing past to future. And while your mind may or may not organize time this way, you can just imagine at this time that your past is to your left and your present is in front of you and your future stretches out to your right, right? Now you can understand even better, the phrases, your past is left behind and your future is right in front of you.

Now notice the interesting parallel between the direction of turning fastening devices like lids and our time organizing by the brain. Is it coincidence that both go to the left for reversing the present status? To undo a lid, for example you turn to the left, lifting and removing the lid, returning the lid's relationship with the jar to what preceded. [*This allows the listener to disconnect from the belief in his mind.*] To go forward, the lid is turned to the right. This holds the status in place, slightly different than time, in that time continues infinitely to the right but the lid stops, keeping the contents intact into the future.

Now imagine this process applying to the four lug nuts holding a tire on a wheel. The tire on the wheel can rotate in either direction infinitely but the lug nuts only tighten to a certain degree, holding the tire on the wheel. Now imagine the tire, any tire, representing a certain belief. [*Place reference to a specific belief here if so desired.*] Have you ever noticed the device that loosens the lug nuts, a lug wrench, rather loosely resembles a question mark? [*Repeated reference to loose sets the stage for applying this loosening. Inviting the person to envision the lug wrench as a question mark deepens the trance state.*] And what if the four lug nuts represent the four parts holding any belief in place, certainty, doubt, being unsure and disbelief. These four must be tight and not loose for any belief, tire, to remain in place. [*The multiple uses of tire, suggests tired of the belief and tired of holding it in place so the grip on the belief loosens.]* And when you see a flat tire you almost always exclaim, no! [*Use 'no!' here to employ the strategy of the 'Meta-yes/ Meta-no' pattern of Bodenhamer (1998), stating 'no' to the old belief and pushing it away.*]

How is it you loosen any belief and the four parts holding it in place? And you know you need to because it left you flat. Well, you begin by applying questions to the four belief support pieces. First we apply questions to our certainty. This loosens the grip it has on our belief but the belief remains in place held by the other three pieces. We continue questioning as our certainty falls away.

The next round of questions wraps around doubt. This process loosens the belief further as questions applied to doubt leads to being unsure. Applying questions to being unsure loosens the belief even more. Questions about certainty leads to doubt leading to being unsure and the next thing your know is disbelief. This last piece just falls away after questions remove the other three. Ready now, the belief is completely loose and free for removing and replacing as desired. Now simply raise the belief suspending it above the ground for a change.

And you know that questioning in the opposite manner made the belief present in the first place. The reverse rotation removes the belief, lefty loosy, righty tighty, naturally enough you know. Once finished placing the new where the old was, knowing the new works better, you almost always let out a resounding, triumphant, yes! (this 'yes!' to accept and embrace the new belief) as you feel the fullness of the new wheel. Notice how it moves you, doesn't it? Now see yourself moving fully and freely to your destination knowing how this will feel … now.

So how do you know when to replace your beliefs? What is the purpose of having beliefs? To provide traction in the movement of your life through all kinds of conditions and all kinds of terrain, down hills and up hills. If the beliefs, tires, you now live on result in your grip slipping, consider applying questions to them to replace them with ones providing better traction allowing you to move surely toward your destination. You will know by the feel of your movement on the pathway.

Can't Imagine That...I Can: *Beliefs About Self-Limitations*

This hypnotic pattern resulted from observing the process that often occurs when a client states that they can't imagine a particular behavior or state. I may ask a client to tell me what they would feel, think or do if they stopped one state and associated into another. Quite often the client will state that they can't imagine what it would be like to feel or act from the different state. But in order to say the feeling or behavior that can't be imagined, it first must be imagined (to some degree) followed by denying the self access to the state. The client is really saying they don't believe they can associate into the state and remain there. So the pattern below addresses the dynamics involved in the imagining and accessing of the process of denying.

One particular client came to see me for issues related to very low self-esteem. This client consistently imagined that others thought negatively about him. He would apply these thoughts to himself, believe them and then feel very depressed. Many irrational thoughts ran through his mind. After he started understanding how he created these negative conclusions about himself, I asked him how he would feel if he no longer felt depressed. He stated that he would feel confident, safe and good about himself. I then asked him what it would be like to feel confident, safe and good about himself. He said that he could not imagine feeling this way.

But I knew that in order for him to identify a state, he had at least to acknowledge it from a dissociated position and that he may, ever so briefly, actually associate into it in order to name it. He may just as quickly dissociate from it but he may quickly go into the state to describe the make-up of it. So the claim of not being able to imagine being in the state cannot be true since the person had to first imagine the state. Staying associated into the resourceful state becomes the challenge.

With the depressed client, I applied the pattern below when he claimed he could not imagine how it would feel to be confident about himself, to experience a sense of safety, and to feel good about himself. He then yielded to the logic about being unable to name a state unless you experience it at least from a dissociated perspective. He could then associate into the states of feeling

86

confident, feeling safe and feeling good about himself. This allowed him to consider new behavioral responses from this collection of states.

These new behavioral responses sustained the positive state just as the previous ones from the state of depressed sustained depression. When this client returned after the interval between sessions he reported significantly reduced depression, increased interaction with others and that he could maintain a feeling of confidence, safety and goodness about himself.

He increased his awareness of his environment by accessing his secondary awareness, which permitted new interpretations of stimuli in his environment and led to new responses. This change in his thinking, emotions and behaviors seemed to be helped by his hearing and processing the hypnotic language pattern that invited him to associate into the desired states of confidence, safety and goodness about himself. The elimination of his pessimism that drove his 'inability' to imagine served as a future leverage point as well. Each time he claimed he could not imagine a new state or behavior I would remind him of his ability to associate into the state just by imagining it and that he knew he could imagine it, couldn't he? With some additional sessions addressing other elements contributing to his depression, this client went on to become free of depression and into a life that he reported to me as being far more satisfying to him.

> **Usually the person who 'can't imagine' really does imagine but believes that he can't operate from the state.**

Very often a person will claim that he just doesn't know how he would feel (state of mind or emotion) if he behaved in a different, more resourceful way. For example, 'How will you feel when you consistently express your wants to others?'. This claim, that the listener just does not know, almost always represents some meaning other than the traditional sense.

Usually the person who 'can't imagine' really does imagine but believes that he can't operate from the state. You can tell if your question prompts a visit to the state by the listener if they pause briefly and shift the direction of their gaze. It is important to elicit the state the person just briefly identified or visited. Point out to the client that you know they just went somewhere and identified a state of mind or emotion. Though briefly experienced, what is the state? Now the issue becomes one of sustaining this state and utilizing it in the future, doesn't it? Once this difference, accessing versus using, gets established, the following pattern becomes applicable:

> Your imagination is one very amazing and elaborate system. It can make anything pop up right out of thin air. Why you can even imagine your imagination, imagine that. It reminds me of being in one of those house of mirrors when you put yourself at just the right angle so you can see a reflection of a reflection of a reflection endlessly in a row within the different mirrors and you can even imagine this.
>
> One of the other interesting features of your imagination is that it can imagine in all five senses. You can imagine tasting a salty food or sweet food and notice the increased salivation, right? You can imagine hearing a favorite piece of music and feel the appeal. You can imagine touching something rough or smooth and notice the feeling in your fingers, they imagine too. What about your smelling sense? Imagine bread baking or chocolate chip cookies baking and then the scent, your nose thinks it knows.
>
> Now the thread running through all these experiences you see is your sight. This thread can be any size or color but you see it accompanies imagined experiences. And we could go really big picture about uncommon common threads running through all, but I'll leave that up to you. See? Get to know it, it is part of you and there for you. And sometimes you say you can't imagine being or acting a certain way. [*The therapist can fill in the specific state or behavior that fits for the client.*] Well, I suggest to you that you do imagine that. How else do you know what it is that you claim you can't imagine. To name it is to know it. So it is not that you can't imagine it because to deny it you first must claim it. Then the real issue is whether you can stay being the way you imagined yourself, right? How is it there and how will it be when you make it here, now?

Imagine you imagine you stay there making it here, pretty sound huh?

Now imagine the many ways you use this and how your imagination is the key gaining entry into any and all. Imagine the possibilities and use because your imagination just starts the process you want to finish, don't you?

It Just Makes Sense: Beliefs about Depression

The words and concept for this pattern came from working with a client who expressed significant depression and relied upon a visual memory to sustain some of the depression. He ran a film in his mind of a particular part of his life that would consistently prompt a feeling of depression. Initial attempts to intervene by altering the content of the memory were ineffective in decreasing his depression. It became apparent that the film itself would need to go away. This would make way for a different film for him to run, which would lead him to a different and more resourceful state of mind-emotion.

The reason for the smoke and fire in the pattern stems from the depressing visual memory he had that seemed to be shrouded in smoke. This gave rise to the idea of burning the memory (film) and having it go up in smoke. Once the smoke rises he could then follow it up to view the process that often occurs at the highest point of visual representational system.

A person usually finds his visual representation of his higher power when he holds his head level and looks up as high as he can.

A person often finds the visual representation of his higher power when he holds his head level and then looks up as high as he can in the center of his visual field. With or without the higher power image though, this visual location very often holds the greatest resources for change and healing.

Once the client had described the visual memory including the smoke effect surrounding it, I began suggesting that he consider burning it to simply rid himself of the memory and its effect. As soon as he expressed interest and curiosity, I began generating this language pattern shown below. During this process the client experienced a strong collection of emotions including tearfulness and an apparent releasing of the old depression-producing memory. After I checked to verify that the memory left him, we began the process of replacing the departed memory with a state that was more consistent with his desired outcome. A reported feeling of relief led to happiness and then to feeling energized. We then explored ways he can view this state collection, feel it and project it into his life to create desired outcomes.

This language pattern exists essentially as a complete induction and change making process, from start to finish. Confusion or dissonance creation is present through the 'good memory about a bad memory' reference. This leads to associating into the memory but then dissociating or suggesting second person awareness to decrease the intensity. Similarity appears with 'all scents' inviting all senses of the listener to rise. Also, 'firing a memory' and 'power of ascent' utilize similarity along with the 'heir' (air) apparent for converting the double meaning into a pathway to change. This pattern proceeds through the big three steps of change by associating the listener into the undesired state, connecting to the desired state and then displaying the desired. Drawing on a spiritual component provides a powerful resource for those oriented in this direction. This language pattern draws from my (BB) visually oriented pattern known as 'How to Take a Bitter Root to Jesus' (1995).

> You can think about a scent and maybe you will notice how it smells. You can choose any of the many scents. If it stinks, you could recall a bad memory but how good is your memory about a bad memory? Maybe it's like when you have a cold and don't smell so good. You may find a vague, foggy stench like old mold on something gone bad and want to send it away, banning the bad memory from your good memory. All scents rise, just think about smoke, visual sense, firing a memory. Then let your fuzzy bad memory scent up to rise higher and higher while the scent becomes fainter and fainter until it rises so high its faints dead away.

Now sending the scent up to the heavens to experience the power of ascent, heaven scent. Notice the new scent, the heir apparent and how it moves you now, doesn't it … provide you with a full bouquet in bloom as you now allow yourself to fully inhale and hearty feeling about what you want to most do now, won't you see, hear, feel, smell and taste the future in the present. You can unwrap it and open it, for use now, wow!

Summary

This chapter examined beliefs, their influence on us and how to effect a change in beliefs through hypnotic language. Beliefs play a crucial role in shaping our perceptions, thoughts, emotions and behaviors. Beliefs set parameters for us and greatly determine one's reality. A person generally behaves in ways that are consistent with beliefs. If beliefs change then perceptions, thoughts, emotions and behaviors follow suit.

Another way of changing beliefs comes through reminding a person of his untapped and infinite potential within, the place of pure potentiality residing in a person's unconscious mind. Here the person can essentially choose any belief desired and then implement it in his life to create a desired outcome.

Beliefs can shift as a result of behaving differently. This different behavior results in a ripple effect that brings new or different outcomes for the actor. The actor then shifts beliefs to ones that are consistent with the new outcome experienced. The principle of cognitive dissonance creates the shift to make beliefs match outcomes because a person needs consistency between beliefs and experiences. The hypnotic language patterns in this chapter invite belief shifts through the three methods identified above.

The Meta-Level Structure of Beliefs

Before leaving beliefs, we felt it appropriate to share some brief remarks from Michael Hall about the meta-level structures involved in belief formation. This information will further add explanation as to why hypnotic language can effect changes in beliefs. We have stated that 'beliefs set parameters for us and greatly determine one's reality'. These 'belief parameters' or 'frames' function as meta-level structures in that they modulate other behaviors. In hypnosis, the client 'reframes' or 're-structures' these belief parameter/frames, hence meta-level beliefs change and subsequent behaviors change with the beliefs.

Michael contributes the following summary of the meta-level structure of beliefs:

> Meta-states provide a specific way to distinguish thought and belief. Overall, thoughts (even complex ones) operate at the primary level as mere representation while beliefs and beliefs-about-beliefs operate at meta-levels.
>
> If you think about 'taking criticism effectively', you have to represent someone giving you a critique. You may think about someone in your past who said something that you felt was critical. You may imagine seeing, hearing, and feeling yourself handling it by listening calmly, asking questions to explore in order to understand, using it as information, etc.

Figure 4:1
The meta-levels of Beliefs

MS: T-F: 'Yes!'
'I validate that!'

@ (about) =

PS: 'I can take criticism offered to me
effectively from someone in the world

Code: T-F: Thoughts-and-feelings, @: about, MS: meta-state, PS: primary state.

But how do you believe in that thought ('I can take criticism effectively.')? You have to move to a higher logical level to think about that thought. Reflexively, your thoughts come back to reflect on your previous thoughts. This puts you at a meta-level to your thoughts-and-feelings about the first level thoughts-and-feelings. Your thoughts no longer refer to something out there in the world, but to something 'in there' in your mind, to your idea of your capacities and skills. Now you're in reference to a concept about conceptual realities. Structurally, a belief involves thoughts about something plus validating, affirming, accepting thoughts about those primary thoughts. This explains why merely repeating an empowering belief statement will not have the same effect as believing an empowering belief statement. [Although habitual repetition will typically elicit a sense of 'confirmation'.]

How do these psycho-logics work? It probably occurs because we typically equate 'familiarity' with 'confirmation'. This gives insight into the structure of disbelief. To disbelieve a statement, we essentially bring thoughts of doubt, unsureness, questions, etc. to bear on the primary thought. 'I have questions about that idea'. Hence, a state of doubt about a state of thought.

From this brief explanation of the meta-level structures of belief, can we not conclude that when we shift beliefs through hypnosis we essentially go to a Meta-level 'no' (or serious doubt) and bring that to bear on the unwanted belief? And, then, we access a Meta-level 'yes' and bring that to bear on the desired belief. Can it be that simple? Maybe so. Maybe so.

Chapter Five

Language Patterns Addressing Time Orientation

'Inasmuch as we can sort and distinguish between *events* that have already occurred, those that now occur, and those that will occur, most humans in most cultures sort for three central *'time' zones*. These show up in the linguistic tenses as well as the temporal tenses of the past, present, and future.'

(p. 174, Hall and Bodenhamer, 1997b, emphasis added)

In what direction do you tend to place your focus: your past, your present or your future? In this chapter, the language patterns address time orientation. By time orientation we mean whether a person pays attention to the past, present or future. Time orientation plays a crucial role in either sustaining problems or solving problems.

I (BB) can give you a recipe for 'depressing' yourself. How? Simply orient your mind primarily towards the *past* and *only* focus on those events that you perceive as causing you hurt. Make sure that you don't look at any good things that happened to you or else you will mess up 'depressing yourself'. And, for certain, don't look at any present good things in your life nor dream a happy future for yourself. In order to depress yourself, just look at all those perceived bad things in your past. Then start talking to yourself about how bad they were and how bad they hurt you. Really juice them up by layering (Meta-stating) negative thoughts upon negative thoughts about those experiences.

The following comes from an actual counseling session I (BB) recently conducted. I asked the client (single female in her 30s) to share with me 'all' that she perceived 'wrong' with her. She gave me all these negative frames:

- I am incompetent in everything.
- I am hopeless.
- I am unhappy.
- I am more depressed than ever.

- I can't maintain a relationship.
- I have trouble motivating myself.
- I feel sick all the time and miserable.
- I can't keep up my hygiene.
- I can't relate to people my age.
- I can't enjoy myself.
- I don't like myself.
- I don't have any self-esteem.
- I don't know what I am going to do next week.
- I can't handle my period. I was worried about that.
- I can't use the bathroom.
- My parents are going to send me to a mental institute.
- I can't handle being by myself.
- I can't stop fidgeting with my hair, my eyebrows, my teeth …
- I don't know how to live.
- I am so irritable.
- Seeing other people prosper irritates me.
- I just want to go to sleep and I can't.
- I can't will myself out of this.
- I am not comfortable with my parents.
- My parents want me out.
- I lived in my apartment by myself and I can't stand it.

Did reading all of these negative frames depress you? She sure knows how to run depression.

I wish I could say that I have made great progress with this client but to date I haven't. Indeed, numerous psychologists, psychiatrists, psychotherapists and counselors have given up on her. I haven't. She has made several serious attempts at suicide. My point in sharing her negative frames: to give them as an example of what can happen when we place our focus totally on bad events in our past and then Meta-state those past memories with negative frames.

> **Because 'time' exists only as a subjective reality, one can use hypnosis to assist a client in 'reframing' his perceptions of the past.**

Because 'time' exists only as a subjective reality, one can use hypnosis to assist a client in 'reframing' his perceptions of the past. In *Time Lining: Patterns for Adventuring in 'Time'* (Bodenhamer and Hall, 1997) we explain:

> ... we have a *nominalization* in the word 'time'. We have a verb (designating a process) which someone has erroneously turned into a static, non-moving noun. Underlying the noun-form of the term we do not have anything that we can put in a wheelbarrow (the NLP test for a nominalization). We have nothing we can see, hear, smell, touch or taste. What does 'time' smell like? Does it have a temperature?
>
> What we have in the word 'time' lies in the realm of an action. First we have *events* happening, then we have our *mental thinking and conceiving* (another process) about those events, which involve our understanding of the relationship between events occurring. *So, 'time' does not have an external referent.* It refers to nothing in the empirical world. It exists as something *invisible*—something in the mind, an abstraction of a higher logical level than 'things ...'
>
> 'Time' then exists as a *conceptual reality*, an understanding of the relationship between events—and not anything actual or literal beyond our nervous system. For some, this high level abstraction about an abstraction (understanding of 'time') takes a while to get used to. We have talked about 'time' as a thing and treated it as external and confused it with 'the clock.' This will also challenge those who operate from a more literal frame of mind and who might not progress much beyond what we call 'the concrete thinking' stage.
>
> In NLP, when we discover an ill-formed map in the form of a nominalization, to recover and understand our meaning, we *denominalize* it ...'
>
> (p.10, emphasis added)

It is this *denominalizing of time* that explains *how* hypnosis works. Hypnosis allows the client to reframe those *seemingly real* past memories so that they now serve in the present as resources rather than as problems.

> **It is this *denominalizing of time* that explains *how*
> hypnosis works. Hypnosis allows the client to
> reframe those *seemingly real* past memories so that
> they now serve in the present as resources rather
> than as problems.**

For instance, a person can focus on her past and some emotional injury that produced a limiting belief and then limit herself from that point forward. But a person can also focus on the past and find a very effective resource that she can apply in the present or future. This same person can make the present her time orientation. She can then notice a necessary ingredient available in the present for the desired outcome she wants to make a reality in the future. What results from this scenario? The person develops a present time orientation that builds up to the creation of a desired future.

Problems and solutions reside within time frames, depending on what time becomes the focus and on what features the person focuses. This determines the 'problems' and 'solutions' that a person invents. These time-oriented language patterns aim to shift the person from problem-producing time orientation to resource-producing time orientation.

Problem-states seem most often to involve a past emotional injury that produces a limiting belief. As long as the person continues to focus on his past, the injury and resulting limiting belief, that person will continue to limit himself in the present and future. The language patterns in this chapter seek to disconnect the listener from a limiting past and connect them to a more resourceful present. Not that the past only holds limitations or problems. The past can also represent a source of solutions to draw from and apply in the present or future.

One can access past memories and disconnect from his perceived negative influence. Next, one can access these past memories and reframe them into learnings and 'bind' them to the present as resources. Then the future can become a blank canvas of opportunities. The listener may be the artist. Hypnotic language addressing 'time' has the possibility of allowing the painter to remember the full spectrum of colors and use any or all colors to paint the desired future. These colors come from the past, the present or the future.

The gestalt perceptual patterns of continuation, dissonance and similarity run through most of these language patterns. These perceptual patterns apply through stopping old continuation, pointing out dissonance and accessing resources consistent with the desired outcome. Then the client utilizes continuation from that point forward. Simplicity as well as figure-ground also play a role in these hypnotic patterns. Simplicity occurs anytime a person goes 'Meta' to his original state. Since Meta-states modify all states beneath them, Meta-stating simplifies the process of managing any situation. Once you reach a Meta-state understanding, responding to a situation becomes simpler because the Meta-state takes care of the details. Pointing out alternatives helps to shift the listener from the old to create a new set of information from which to draw for making a desired present and future.

The Bubble of Is: The Benefits of Living in the Present

I developed this language pattern while thinking about 'time' and one's 'place' of residence as past, present or future. Then I asked myself the question, 'how do we create fear or anxiety?' In order to experience fear, a person must place herself in the future and then imagine possible negative outcomes (a Meta-stating process). Producing fear about the present moment cannot happen. Fear can only revolve around what might happen, but has not (see the language pattern, 'almost') yet happened. Even if the feared event happens, then fear is only sustained by what may occur next. Fear is not about what is but what may become of what is.

> **Producing fear about the present moment cannot happen. Fear can only revolve around what might happen, but has not yet happened.**

As an example, imagine yourself confronted by a possible thief. He has a gun pointed at you and asks for your money. In order to create 'fear' you will probably see yourself (a created image of the future) emptied of your wealth and fear that by saying to yourself something like, 'I worked hard for my money. What will I do without it?'. Or, you may very well see yourself being shot and create fear and/or panic by taking the imagined image of your being shot and generate words that make meaning of it like, 'I am too young to die!' or 'I don't want to die!' In either case, your fear results from a *perceived negative future*. You cannot experience a fear of death without imagining your death, and the implications of it for your future. If the fear of death occurs about the present, you are already dead.

Let's consider this point further. The reference made to 'being' shot, hurt, violated, etc., bases itself on the future, not the present. Even if shot, the fear/anxiety results from what may happen as a result of being shot, not the being shot. In other words, what does being shot mean? Maybe it means I may die or be permanently disabled. But these meanings draw upon possible future outcomes, not the present since neither of these outcomes are actually happening in the now. The gun pointing at the victim may or may not be bad. For the victim to determine the pointing gun is bad, the victim would need to imagine a negative outcome beyond the moment.

Oddly, it seems that focusing on not having some specific resource keeps you from accessing that resource.

In addition to generating fear by imagining a negative future, a person may also experience fear or other undesirable states by residing in the past. Focusing on the past and what one supposedly got deprived of actually results in self-deprivation in the present, since the missing resource and all resources remain continually available in the present. When an unpleasant event happened in the past and it becomes your sole focus in the present, it invites you to then also imagine your future void of this desired outcome. In fact, if you don't imagine your future or present being void of this resource, then unpleasant emotions disappear. Oddly, it seems that focusing on not having some specific resource keeps you from accessing that resource. Unpleasant emotion-states result from this process of living in a self-limiting past and/or future, rather than the all-things-possible 'is' of the moment.

It may be valid to say that negative or limiting emotions, such as depression or anger, can only be generated in the current moment. But drawing on the past or future can complicate the negative emotions about the present by adding Meta-layers to the limiting state. In order to produce a Meta-layer of unpleasant emotion-state in the moment, we must first step out of 'is' in either direction, past or future. It seems a person can live in a sort of potentially protective bubble of 'is'. When a person lives exclusively in the 'is' bubble, then all is available. The person living in the bubble of 'is' possesses awareness of only what is happening, not what has or may happen. When living out of 'is', the person only knows what is not. Living in the present permits effective decisions and movement toward desired outcomes.

Desired outcomes are what you want your future 'is' to be when you get there. The desired outcome can be determined while remaining within 'is'. Actually, desired outcomes utilize 'is' by imagining constructive applications of 'is' in the future. This creates a powerful motivating loop. Think about a project you may currently be working on and imagine it flopping in the future. How does this affect motivation in the 'is' of the present? Motivation only increases if you draw upon an away-from or avoiding strategy. But this strategy still requires converting the undesired into positive action. Some of the energy gets lost in the transfer.

Now envision the project you work on resulting in a wonderful outcome. What sort of energy infusion results? A very fine invigorating loop develops as each desired outcome and 'is' feed each other positive energy making them grow stronger. 'Is' remains ever flexible for your use as you see fit. So this hypnotic pattern holds as its purpose reminding the listener that remaining within the 'is' allows an absence of fear or other uncomfortable emotion-states and a full awareness and experience of what is.

Reaching the goal of the language pattern relies on most of the gestalt perceptual principles. Simplicity gets addressed by actually simplifying time orientation, making this more appealing to the individual. And the bubble of the 'is' concept appeals to the need for closure. This pattern actually guides the listener into a better state. From that positive state the pattern displays the method so the person will naturally feel motivated to use the new tool for sustaining the benefit—continuation after elevation to a more resourceful Meta-state.

The client came into the session complaining of anger and ultimately fears of losing self-worth. A situation had occurred at work in which his supervisor treated him in a way that felt disrespectful to him. The supervisor had transferred my client to another department within the company. The supervisor rationalized the transfer rather than honestly owning his own self-serving motives.

The employees in this new department worked very well together. The other workers had created a light atmosphere with much joking and an overall enjoyable work experience. But the client deprived himself of the present, new atmosphere, by focusing on the past and how his self-worth became diminished. He then saw this negative frame continuing into the future. The client, by fixing upon the past, deprived himself of enjoying the present and thus experienced unpleasant emotional states. While this example involves a client living in the past, this pattern seems very effective for reducing anticipatory anxiety. (Is there any kind of 'anxiety' other than 'anticipatory' anxiety?)

> James, I know your past supervisor treated you in a way that you feel was unfair. And I realize that this leads to you feeling angry, hurt and like he may think you are dumb [*all his labels elicited in conversation prior to the language pattern*]. But I also wonder how dumb he must be to think you may be that dumb. And I wonder what you will feel like when you get past the past moving you into the present that you can now open to find that you in fact work with other people that you feel good being around, sort of like a nice complete circle.
>
> And in fact when you live in the *present* it *is* sort of like living in a bubble, the bubble of is. [*While describing this bubble, I motion with my hands a circle about twice the size of a basketball*

right in front of the client.] In this protective bubble of *is* you get to enjoy what *is* happening now and you like what *is* happening now where you work, don't you? And when you leave the bubble of *is*, you don't know what *is*, only what is not and you lose what you enjoy then don't you?

So in order to really find and feel the change from past to present *is* good for you, you need to live in the present, feeling it now like you like. And how do you feel when you remain in the bubble of *is* closing out the past leaving you with only awareness of what *is* and what you want to continue, won't you now?

After this pattern, James reported feeling a deeper understanding of the importance and benefit of living in the present. He stated that he now sees the connection between living in the present and feeling good. He reported feeling as though the change to another department was truly a blessing for him that he now can enjoy. (Hence, hypnosis, as does all successful therapy, reframed the problem state into a resource state.) This pattern itself, like 'is', is very flexible and can be molded to fit thought patterns that generate anxiety about the future just as easily as extracting the listener from the past to enjoy the fruits of the present.

Next: The 'Next' Step in Obtaining Your Desired Outcome

In this word pattern I utilize the action-compelling word 'next' to propel the listener toward his desired outcome. A 'next' step plays in every strategy or process a person uses to realize a goal. A problem occurs when we allow our 'nexts' to lead us away from our desired outcome. ('Next' functions as an ordinal presupposition in Milton model language.) Very often we go astray because we focus on the past rather than drawing from our vision of our desired outcome. The past gets superimposed on the present resulting in history repeating itself.

Very often we go astray because we focus on the past rather than drawing from our vision of our desired outcome. The past gets superimposed on the present resulting in history repeating itself.

The words in this pattern draw from the vast resources within our unconscious mind obtained by living and experiencing life. Just having in mind a desired outcome presupposes that there exists a way to 'think', 'feel' and 'do' in order to bring about the desired outcome. 'And what will you know after you achieve this? If you will know this then you can know this now, can't you?' A person can essentially retrace her future back to her present by stepping on the sequence of 'next' stepping stones in reverse. A person can draw on the awareness that will be present in her future and let it guide her movements from the 'here and now' to the 'there' and 'then'.

The language pattern presented uses continuation in reference to what will be consistent with the desired outcome and suggesting the listener continue it 'now'. Also, dissonance comes into play along with simplicity and similarity. Similarity occurs in the fourth line with 'here...this...now.' The dissonance happens when time orientation gets twisted by asking the listener to go into the past, the future and then come back to the present. The simplicity concept applies by removing complicating steps in the present and simply asking the person to focus on the outcome she desires in the future. It's like mind backtracking (Bodenhamer and Hall, 1997) but starting from the desired state to identify the path in the present that will lead you to the desired future.

> Now you know what you do not want to do and, more importantly, you know what you do want to do. You can look in your past to notice all the steps, one after another, a series of *nexts* leading you up to here ... this ... now that you know what you want, look into your future and see yourself thinking, feeling and doing as you want. See the outer edges of your future self and moving toward the center notice the stronger deeper awareness of what and how you want to be then feeling this now notice what your *next* step is in making your future happen now. What will be your *next next* and ... so ... on ... until ... you create a clear path of *nexts* leading you right up to ... what and how you want to be ... now? And now simply allow your mind to inform all of you what to do *next*.

Bingo: Accessing the Place Before it All Began to Make it All Different Now.

As a child I (BB) use to love to spin myself around and around faster and faster until I got so 'drunk' that I would fall down. This hypnotic language pattern amounts to spinning the person's time orientation around and around until they lose orientation. Because the brain seeks equilibrium, this gives the hypnotherapist opportunity to point the listener in the direction of the agreed upon outcome.

I (JB) draw from a well-known game called bingo for the metaphor. The double meaning of the phonological ambiguity '*B-4/before*' provides the phrase for shifting the client. 'Before' fits the category of prepositions in the English language and serves as a temporal preposition/presupposition in NLP.

> **Prepositions represent a dissociated perspective. The very word, pre-position, infers the previous position to the current one.**

Prepositions represent a dissociated perspective. The very word, pre-position, infers the previous position to the current one. Prepositions allow time travel because of their very nature. Prepositions in general and 'before', in particular, dissociate the listener from her current position making free movement and choice possible. 'Before' becomes a vehicle of time travel in this pattern and transports the person back in time to the point 'before' any other 'befores'—the conceptual 'void', where nothing yet is, and then to the place where any and all things are possible, the totality of secondary awareness. No limiting beliefs exist here, that is in the 'void'. Once associated into the place of all things possible (the 'void'), I then transport the person forward to the present with this new awareness of 'all things are possible'. From the present, I Future Pace the listener by pointing them to their future again using the timeless word-concept, 'before'.

The start of this pattern should come off the listener's launching pad. By this, I mean launch the pattern from the specific issue, concept or belief that the listener presents to you. Once the client provides a time orientation statement, utilize her statements to begin your pattern. The 'it' in the pattern vaguely refers to the 'problem' or stuck spot presented by the client, the client's misconception. In some sense all personal limitations result from misuse of time since there is a time in which all things exist as possibilities, actually always (see 'The Bubble of Is' language pattern in this section). When we do not draw from our 'Is of Possibilities' we live from a highly restricted belief time frame and, therefore, lay the groundwork for personal distress.

> It reminds me of those floating, whirling white ping-pong balls within the vacuum machine in the bingo hall. Looking into the bin noticing how your eyes are able to follow moving [*I intentionally skip here to induce more dissonance and dissociating—subtly refer to moving to another state. I could place the word* objects *here but want to avoid the possible double meaning with this to reduce reluctance*] and distinguishing an individual white ball from the blurred mass. Now knowing only one from the many and in particular the one numbered B-4. [*Symbolically, the collection of bingo balls represent secondary awareness while the single one, 'B-4', that I focus the client on constitutes primary awareness. I use this to subtly remind the mind of both the conscious and unconscious.*]

> This is especially interesting because what was *before* and what will be next as the last next was *before* and *before* is timeless because what is *before* you is both the past and the future you know, and you can glimpse behind to see what is left *before* you. How many *befores* do you step over counting your way back to *before* the first one? And what do you call the time *before* any of your *befores* begin?

> Feeling this ... now ... see and feel the future is right *before* you to realize you can see how the past was left behind while the future is right in front of you want to do what is right now, don't you see how it stretches out already? Your future does not know your past, how will you tell it to be? What will happen next? If you know how you will be in your future and you know it will be good for you what are you waiting for now. ... Feel this now.

Future Perfect: Eliminating the Limiting Influence of the Past

This time twisting pattern seeks to clarify, then confuse and then clarify through time dissonance. The person first associates to the problem state; second, they dissociate from the problem state; and, third they associate into the resource state. This moves the client from a state of limitation to a resourceful state.

Simplicity occurs by removing the 'cloud of the past' from the client's present. Similarity occurs with the words: 'superimposing', 'through' and 'undesirable presents'. Continuation naturally happens as each pattern invokes continuation because we just keep going on the track we get set upon. Closure contributes to the process when the person's time orientation is first disrupted and then reassembled to a point of closure about the future.

> **A person often generates a problem when observing the present through the eyes of the past.**

The conceptual principle here involves the notion that a person often generates a problem when observing the present through the eyes of the past. This leads to habitual responses to similar stimuli resulting in history repeating itself. The goal of the pattern is to remove the veil of the past from the present allowing awareness of only what is happening in the present. Removing the veil from the past gives the client the ability to form more constructive and resourceful choices in which to bring about her desired outcome.

> When you think about each time you felt bad, don't you find that you had to live in the past? When you experience distress it always seems to result from experiencing the past in the present. The present event may not actually make for distress but superimposing the past on the present, and this really is a super imposition, brings about an ineffective choice because of the blurred awareness. How upsetting it must be to force yourself to observe *what is* through… the cloud of *what was.* Imagine how clear your vision will be when seeing the present, only. And just how will you know when you do this? Well, you will notice only all choices and possibilities and how good this will feel.

And while I just stated that the only way to feel bad is to see the present through the past, you are correct when you notice it is possible to feel bad when imagining the future. But just how do you accomplish this feat? To accomplish this you must go into the future believing some undesirable present remains with you. And you can take back and return undesirable presents making it before. So essentially, you take the present into the future, which makes it the past and then see the present, which was the future, through the past, which was the present, you know.

So still you can only feel bad by experiencing the present through the past and you can feel good knowing only the present and how you want it to be in the future. When this thought *passes* and *becomes the past*, clearing the way for *the present* future what do you notice freely and clearly *now*? Only tune this in and experience this for this is all you need to experience to make your future experience what you desire. What is what you will do... *now*?

The Other Side of the Mirror: *Shifting Focus from Past to Future*

This pattern involves more of a visual approach to intervening in the person's time orientation. Similarity comes into play with 'looking forward to the future' (2nd paragraph). The pattern encourages some dissonance by use of the word 'notice' on a repeated basis. This also serves to dissociate the person further from the past orientation. Simplicity and continuation take place because each pattern simplifies a process and assumes the person will just naturally continue the new, more effective, process.

It seems that one of the main ways a person feels bad emotionally is to look at the present through the past. Doing this is sort of like using a mirror to look at the present, all you see is what's behind you and then mistake it for what is before you. Of course the next thing you know is just what you knew before so history repeats repeats itself.

Now I wonder, and you may wonder also, what will happen when you step through the mirror? Stepping through the mirror immediately removes the past view and now all you know is the present and the future, you look forward to the future, you know. And looking forward to the future just what of the infinite possibilities do you notice and what do you want to *notice* so that you can use now to serve *notice* to yourself to *notice* now what you can use now to make into the future you want then now.

And now just *notice* how and what new ideas come into your mind in the present about the future. Feel these ideas become a fuel that propels you toward them and the closer you get the more you feel propelled toward them so you just naturally want to move closer and closer, don't you now?

Forecast: Creating a Rewarding Future for the Present

This language pattern relies on certain principles of human nature. Each of us exhibits somewhat predictable thoughts and behaviors. Knowing these predictable thought processes and behaviors gives the hypnotherapist the necessary awareness of cognitive processes. This knowledge permits redirecting the client's thoughts/ behaviors towards a more productive purpose.

> **The snapping of fingers in this hypnotic pattern demonstrates a predictable principle: people give attention to events that stand out.**

Just after beginning the pattern, the therapist holds his hand out to his side and snaps his fingers. The listener will naturally look at the therapist's fingers that he just snapped. The snapping of fingers in this hypnotic pattern demonstrates a predictable principle: people give attention to events that stand out. The pattern then invites the listener into a trance because the therapist now gets the attention or focus of the listener.

Once in a trance, the listener is then guided to apply the principle of noticing events that stand out within the client's time orientation. Once you have the client attending to the standout events, you can then direct the client's attention wherever you wish (NLP pacing and leading). The person can then do what amounts to figure-ground reversal with her time frame. She can notice the present or future or positive rather than negative events or resourceful rather than limiting beliefs. The last half of this pattern shifts the time orientation from past to future encouraging the listener to 'cause' or predict the future by utilizing the present in a way that is consistent with the future.

After explaining the process of how a person disconnects from useful resources, the listener receives an invitation to reclaim past resources that the client has forgotten. Confusion and appeal to dissonance occurs frequently in the last several sentences making use of humor as well.

Piaget's concept of transductive logic also serves a crucial role in making this pattern effective, as does the either—or style of thinking. Frequently, when an aversive event happens, a person will mistakenly believe that the state or resource they used is the cause of the aversive event. The state or resource then gets put away because the person comes to believe the state is 'bad'. Sometimes modifying the state or resource, not either–or use, can create solutions.

> Some processes in life are truly predicable. Cause and effect can be known before they repeat. If you hear a noise to your left [*extend your right hand to your far right and snap your fingers*], you naturally look there for the source. Upon hearing a noise to your right [*Extend your left hand to your far left and snap your fingers*], you naturally look there for the source. These reactions are quite predictable. You could easily forecast them and, in fact, cause them by creating noise in a certain direction knowing the response will be directing attention toward the noise.

> If your past makes noise it diverts attention from the present and future. When your future makes noise it draws you toward it in order to find out what's up. In the past, we sometimes made choices about putting some behaviors or states out of the lineup and in storage. You know only two reasons exist for removing behaviors or states from active roles. They either did not bring the desired result or brought an undesirable result. Yes, these are different and reflect moving toward or away from certain outcomes.

> You do not use a behavior or state that misses the mark nor will you use one that creates aversive circumstances. Each of these strategies is context dependent of course. The state may

be useful somewhere else and later it may bring different consequences. You will know by assessing what is different in the present than in the past.

Using forecasting inability these ineffective behaviors get placed in storage as if the weather is identical each day. If no rain falls *one* day do you sell your umbrella? When is the time to bring them out of storage? However, the events of the past sometimes continue exerting influence and interfere with accurate vision of the present becoming the future.

It is important to see the present and the future for what they are and can be instead of what they were. Imagine your past is in North Dakota and your future in Kansas. Well, you'd want to forgo Fargo and take a peak at Topeka. What if you were going to live in Belair? What would you do when you got there to get around and not be square? Whatever you do, do not stare just dare to compare.

Appearances matter you know, and what is the matter with your appearances? Change the matter and change the appearance. How are you and how are you not? Consider reversing the have with the have not. The cart runs backwards when the horse is behind. Further, the horse can't see very well as the view is obstructed, you see the order you need now don't you? Place it and get what you want but make sure it's thoroughly done. What you want forecasts the future. Your current focus is what will be now and then living up to the forecast.

Nowhere: Overcoming Discouragement by Remembering Resources

Very often certain words lend themselves to flexibility that allows the word to stretch which will then lead to results that are opposite in meaning to the original form. As we have previously mentioned, the category of words in the English language known as prepositions create a conceptual pre-position. What an interesting concept. Prepositions tend to lead the speaker or listener to dissociate from a current state to a state previously held—that is, her pre-position. Experiment with prepositions and notice how they provide opportunities to dissociate.

Prepositions tend to lead the speaker or listener to dissociate from a current state to a state previously held—that is, her preposition.

This concept of varying some words slightly to yield a very different meaning applies to the word 'nowhere'. Utilizing similarity as the springboard, 'nowhere' gets divided into two words, 'now here'. What a difference between 'nowhere' and 'now here'. This difference serves as the resource for altering a person's sense that she is going 'nowhere', to, she is currently residing 'now here'. The effect brings the person back to being within herself, here and now, allowing access to her rich resources. The usual reliance on continuation and egocentrism occurs at the end of the pattern. The pattern leads the person to apply the new and resourceful 'here and now' perspective to her life.

> *Nowhere*, now this word and the concept you think about associated with it can lead to very interesting implications. Thinking about the word *nowhere* makes it *somewhere*, at least in your mind, and separating the *now* makes it now *here* instead of *nowhere*, you see, sort of opposites? Amazing what a little space can do.

> So what is *nowhere*? When you look for it you go *somewhere*. It's sort of like that rainbow thing. Every time you get *where* you thought it was you see it still some distance from you. So no matter where you go it's not *nowhere* because you are there and you can't be *nowhere*. When you don't go to it, going *nowhere*, you are *now here*. While pursuing it is to lose it and just letting it be is to be *now here*.

> So what is *now here* within you and what is *nowhere* to be found? Now here this, all your resourceful, positive emotions are *now here* along with all possibilities. So don't go off to *nowhere* looking for *what is... now here* and feel this, don't you...begin imagining ways you can use *what is here now*?

Glass Floor: Recovering and Healing Lost Parts of Self

This hypnotic pattern amounts to an induction that takes the person from his present to his past for the purpose of resolving an old issue. The early lines begin suggesting dissonance through various situations. This loosens the hold of the current state, which may result in dissociating the client from their problem. The listener can then access a state of reassurance, comfort or some similar state. Following this, a reversal of figure and ground occurs by injecting the old wound from the past (the figure drawing attention) with new, adult resourceful beliefs (ground that needs to come to the forefront, or conscious mind from the unconscious to provide the solution.)

The process occurs from a rather dissociated, objective perspective, i.e. 'a story removed'. 'Removed' in this case also draws boundaries around the wound and readies it for what amounts to a removal. Injecting secondary awareness into the limited primary awareness from childhood allows the injured part of the person to grow up. This equates to re-imprinting or developing new beliefs/identity from alternative responses imagined in the past.

Invoking the saving by Christ also provides additional support, security and comfort. Naturally, only include the Christ reference when speaking to Christians. For non-Christians you may choose to pace their beliefs by utilizing their spiritual resources for re-imprinting. The last few lines contain further distancing from the past beliefs and encourage use of the new in the future.

> When you think about your collection of memories, as you can, it is interesting to know that each experience is unique and can never be experienced the same way twice. Have you ever watched a movie a second time seeing it differently from the first? What about watching the second half of a movie first? Then watching the first half you know the solutions the actors have yet to discover. How different than the actors you feel knowing.
>
> Each time we recall a memory the experience is slightly different yet is about the same experience. It is almost like recalling an original memory is like standing on a glass floor above the event looking down on it out of the flow of the actual experience yet privy to all the information within. And as you view the old experience or memory looking down from above you can know you were wanting to know more then and now…creating a whole new awareness and belief as you look from above down to the event, a story removed.

Now injecting your wisdom into then. After all, this is what kept this memory waiting in your mind. It just wants what you know now to transform then ... freeing the memory to become what it intended to be, feel it grow up now ... knowing all along you would come back and free the mistaken memory, how Christ-like you know, when you really think about it, the savior. But the memory was not really mistaken because it knew you would know how to inform and inject it right... to be free becoming part of the complete whole, feeling the fullness and using to fulfill its purpose now and in the future you can see full of possibilities.

Sometimes when we change we say we no longer know who we are but it really means we are no longer who we were knowing full well who we most truly are now and will be feeling this deeply or maybe even deeper knowing how you can live this ... n-o-w always.

Here and There Now and Then: Tapping the Unconscious Mind's Resources

A total inversion of time and awareness takes place in the first line of this pattern. I accomplish this by asking the listener to become aware of what he is not aware of. This immediately invokes secondary awareness or the unconscious mind. The use of the simple yet powerful temporal presuppositions 'here' and 'there', refers to content or resources. Time travel happens with the experiencing of the temporal presuppositions 'now' and 'then'. Going back and forth serves to confuse and dissociate the person allowing further awareness of freedom of choice. The last section asks the listener to consider what he needs from his unconscious mind and then brings it into his conscious mind for use in the present.

You know what you experience at this very moment but do you know what you do not experience at this very moment? What is *here* in the *now* and what is there in the *then*. Of course then can represent past or future, any time other than *now*, you know? So you know what you have and use *now*, your primary awareness you might call it. Then you can shift to your secondary awareness you might call it. This secondary awareness knows *there* and *then*, all other possibilities.

Your secondary awareness knows and can go to *there* and *then*, making it *here* and *now* for your primary awareness, you know? What state or style or resource does your primary awareness know is missing for the most effective results? What and how do you need to be *here* and *now* that is *there* and *then*...using this *here* and *now* what do you primarily experience? You can *now* hear this, *here* and *now* k-n-o-w *there* and *then*, can't you use this *then* and *now*?

Memories From Your Future—Backpacking:
Releasing Ineffective Childhood Teachings

We place the emphasis here on the natural human condition of transition from childhood into adulthood. Each person receives many teachings from his parents. From these parental teachings we form our values and beliefs. While the family may operate from these values and beliefs, this same collection may not function very well in our adult life.

Along with reference to the backpack of values and beliefs—a sort of family heirloom collection—reference to the emotional state and corresponding physical sensation invokes a deeper and more effective trance. This serves to associate the person into the beliefs and states he wants to eventually leave in the past. The language pattern then utilizes the extended metaphor of unpacking the *backpack*, shifting emotional states and beliefs to then *pack back* up the *backpack* (phonological ambiguity).

The contents of the backpack now include consistent (similarity and simplicity concepts) items in keeping with effective outcomes. This consistent collection then receives a boost of strength by including reference to mental-emotional states. Future Pacing or continuation plays out at the end of the pattern. Some confusion or dissonance occurs with use of 'backpack' and 'pack back'. This also subtly refers to the past as being behind the person in her mental time organization.

The last paragraph utilizes the Ericksonian tag question 'aren't you' to drive home the point. In utilizing tag questions, we seek to direct the primary awareness (conscious mind) to the tag question

115

at the end of the sentence. At the same time, we hope that the suggestion included in the sentence prior to the tag question will slip right into secondary awareness (unconscious mind). You understand, don't you?

As you think about your memories from your *past*, you may begin getting an emotion and physical sensation about these memories. Maybe the *past* unpleasant memories *weigh you down*. You may associate an unpleasant emotion with these heavy memories.

Perhaps these memories feel like a full *backpack*, straps across your shoulders. Now taking the *backpack off* and opening the flap, you may choose to *unpack* the entire contents noticing how it *lightens*. Now you may chose to simply *backpack* or *pack back* those useful memories that proved helpful *then* and now.

You only *want certain learnings from the past* that assist and have good purpose. Notice how they naturally seem...to *fit together*. And you feel them, knowing their presence, they remain with you, intangible and safely secluded from others, only you know of them. They remain proof proof. *Feeling different* than before, *excluding limiting memories* making room only for memories that convert onto practical assistance.

And the word and concept of memory apparently suggests recalling the past. It may seem the only place memories come from. Yet, *you can see* and experience memories from your future. You can now imagine how you *want your future* and remember your future *now...* and then using your good memory remembering the tools you will want in your backpack anticipating reaching your goal, aren't you *now*? Feeling and knowing you can use your memory of your future to choose *now* how to do what will make your future the memory you want so that all present actions are in keeping with the future memory you want, aren't you?

Past Past: *Moving Beyond the Past into the Present*

> **Relationships often succeed because the couple focuses primarily on the present.**
>
> **By focusing on the present, this permits the healthy couple to aim towards a more mutually desired future (a Meta-State).**

Here we focus on releasing the past in order to have a satisfying present and future. Relationships often succeed because the couple focuses primarily on the present. By focusing on the present, this permits the healthy couple to aim towards a more mutually desired future (a Meta-state). Thus, holding on to the grudges of the past will not even exist in these Meta-stated thought processes. The couple does not expend useless effort in jumping to conclusions from pre-conceived limiting beliefs. Such behavior only serves to harm the relationship.

This couple lives in the present while aiming towards a mutually fulfilling future. The theme in this story is: make the prophecy the one you most desire by utilizing only the present to convert it into the desired future. The past is irrelevant unless you refuse to learn from it and to release it.

> Once there was a man who lived in a land far away from here. This land was rather backward and underdeveloped. But a simple pleasure comes from this backward underdeveloped style. The people just work and lead a life of simple ways, uncomplicated, you know? This actually allows the people of this land so far away from here to just pay attention to what is most important, and they know what is most important. They pay attention to what they know, you know?
>
> So in this land far away the people value relationships a lot. One particular man owned a house and some land. He worked very hard on his land making wonderful foods grow with great expertise. He partakes of some and sells some. In his spare time he plays music, just a simple wind instrument producing a very soothing sound. However, this one man knows something is missing from his life. He wants very

117

much to find and make a life with a woman companion. He spends many days and nights wanting, wishing and longing for someone to come into his life and fill the missing piece.

One evening near dusk while he plays his wind instrument he sees the vague outline of a figure approaching him. As this figure gets closer he can tell this is a woman who seems to be about his age. She moves slowly and gracefully. As she nears, she greets him and inquires about his music. She expresses much appreciation for its soothing nature. She sits down and they begin talking. They talk well into the night and begin to see the first signs of daylight. Reluctantly they part but vow to meet the same evening. Sure as dusk approaches so does the woman to this man making music. They talk for hours and begin a tradition of visiting each evening.

This man in this land so far away from here decides to ask this woman to marry him. She embodies all that he wishes for. She easily agrees and joyously marries and moves in to start their life together. The days go by living in bliss. They share a fine compatibility and harmony. This life seems it will go on forever. But with the passing days this man grows curious about his wife's past. While they talked for hours, days and months it always involved sharing current thoughts and feelings and future wants. They painted their future together using their present.

One day he begins inquiring about his wife's past. He asks about her parents, siblings and past experiences of her life. Initially, she expresses great reluctance to discuss her past. He believes her reaction indicates something from her past must need concealing, so he presses on all the more. The more he presses the more she displays hesitation and begins distancing herself from him to prevent the standoff. He continues chasing what he more and more strongly believes simply has to be seriously wrong about her past.

Her refusal to discuss only fuels his fire to get hotter and hotter. The heat and distance from the heat increases. Now dread of interaction replaces the chase followed by her sudden disappearance, never to return. *He had no present with her past and now has no future with her present. All this because he did not get past the past.*

Root Problem: *Reconnecting to Your Deepest, Truest Awareness*

The story told in this pattern invites the listener to travel within him from primary awareness to his secondary awareness. By describing the character in the story as traveling from the city to the wilderness, away from all civilization into the deep woods, I propose to take the client from primary awareness to secondary awareness. The story seeks to motivate the client by a building up of a state of distress and then directing the client towards his outcome as he searches for a remedy to his distress. The remedy exists metaphorically deep in the woods and coming from a particular tree.

The pattern seeks to install a classic NLP 'Propulsion System' within the client. The 'state of distress' serves as the 'Away From' value that pushes the client away from pain and towards a solution. The 'search for a remedy' serves as the 'Towards Value' that pulls the client towards the resolution of his distress.

Trance inducing details about the visual surroundings invite the listener to associate into the story and then travel into his unconscious mind (the 'woods'). Similarity, continuation and various states of mind-emotion along with the states corresponding physical sensation combine to pave the path, shifting the listener from distress to solution.

Similarity occurs with the use of the words, 'knot' (suggesting the negation of the problem-producing state), 'solution' and 'root.' 'Root' invites the listener to go deeper within himself to connect to the root, or origin, of the troubling state. Since the story is a metaphor, the concept of similarity encourages the listener to place the story and its message in category that is similar to his real life issues. The listener is again associated into the problem, dissociated from the problem and then associated into a solution state. Since a person naturally perpetuates whatever state he occupies, the solution state will naturally get applied to the issues that need tending in his or her life-continuation.

This story begins in a large city. Many large buildings sur-
round the center of town and little space can be seen between
these tall structures. This restricts the view. Most of the downtown consists of buildings, dark pavement and sidewalks
with very few, sparsely spaced trees.

One particular person works in this large city with the large,
tall buildings. One particular day he is not feeling well. You
know the feeling; something seems just off kilter, sort of out
of balance. While internally searching he realizes the nature
of the ailment. Once recognizing the issue, the realization
then trips a memory of what a very insightful person once
told him about the solution. Fortunately his memory links the
two together, very convenient. He remembers hearing about
a special root in the wilderness yielding the remedy. He now
sets out on a journey from the city to the wilderness to partake of the remedy.

As he begins traveling from downtown toward the outskirts
of the city he notices the pattern of diminishing building size
and frequency. It almost seems an exchange program because
as the buildings decrease the space between them increases
and more trees come out to play. Now, also houses begin
appearing as the transition continues to include people's
dwellings.

Traveling further, fewer and fewer houses can be seen as he
moves beyond the dwellings, while more and more trees and
space occupy the view of the land. No sidewalks can be seen
now as so few people live here —there is no need. Looking in
the rearview mirror he realizes that all truths exist back there,
then wondering what truths he will choose to live in the
future.

Propelling forwards along the road, moving further and further from the city toward the wilderness, soon the trade is
nearly complete. Now just a road weaves among the wilderness of all the trees and natural space. Eventually the road
comes to an end but his journey continues. Stepping out of his
car, he begins walking along a small but clear path. On each
side, a variety of trees, flowers, vines and other growth frame
his path. Knowing all the while just what he seeks, he takes
note of the different trees and their distinctive bark. This rem-
edy-yielding tree also has a distinctive knot. So he will know
when he is at the right place because of the knot.

Strolling along the path he continues observing for the particular tree with the particular bark with the particular root that yields the solution. He immediately knows when he reaches the antidote tree.

This is the most amazing tree. Part of the root system grows deeply underground, because some of the roots need the warmth and nourishment available under the cover of the ground. But another part of the root system grows in such a way as to protrude just above ground level running parallel to the soil. It resembles a partially buried cable. This way it receives both the warmth and nutrition of the earth while meeting the different sustenance needs through partially exposing its roots.

Further, if any of the exposed section of the roots experiences nicks, the tree immediately regenerates the absent portion. It just stays healthy this way. Standing in awe, the respectful visitor bends down collecting a small sample of the exposed root. The nature of the tree is such that only a small portion of the potion will resolve all. It is quite concentrated. Taking and consuming he immediately begins to feel the solution circulating within. He knows, he feels.

After pausing to further absorb the external and internal peace, he gradually begins his journey, going to other places he knows he wants to be. He will retrace his path that brought him to the wilderness going from there, yet the sights and sounds will feel differently from here on. And if he feels the need to return he will now remember his way. What he now knows is the path provides the solution.

Your First Initial, the Point When It All Began:
Accessing Your Purpose Prior to Limiting Beliefs

The contents of this language pattern rely heavily on similarity and dissonance along with continuation. The use of the words 'sign', 'point', 'line', 'initial' and 'write' represent examples of similarity. Dissonance gets created when referring to a 'different self' in the first paragraph and the reference in the third paragraph of putting 'two and two together.'

The second sentence of the first paragraph applies the process of dissociating the listener from his current state. The use of time orientation asks the listener to shift in time within his mind going back to before his memory of any events in his life. The freedom to create from scratch what he now chooses becomes available. The words invoke auditory, visual and kinesthetic senses to enrich and deepen the intervention.

> You know how to sign your name and what name to sign. And your name is just a sign representing your self. You recognize your name in writing and you even turn your head when you hear your name said out loud by someone else. It is sort of interesting and surprising when you see your name in writing but you know it was not you who wrote it, someone of similar name but different self. You have a similar response when someone who you do not see right away calls your name.
>
> How do you know if it is you who they call? You check your memory banks very quickly to see or hear if you can find a match for what you see or hear now. Is the voice familiar, or do the lines seem like ones you feel familiar with? You know, sometimes others ask you to write just your initials instead of your full name.
>
> Some circumstances call for you to put all three initials and sometimes you just need to put two. If you have a spouse you put two and two together. Either way you go these letters serve as your sign. And please do not begin considering all the possible meanings for the word sign here. This may lead you back in time to when you write your first initial which comes off as rather redundant, your first initial. But what is before your first initial? Yes, the point before it all begins. The writer is known as the author and you are the author authority. Now you can make it write... what... you...want... to. S-e-e?

Wake UP: Using Your Present to Steer to Your Future

This short induction and metaphor invites the listener to consider the role that her time orientation plays in affecting how effectively she directs her life. Drawing upon similarity ('wake'), simplicity (I do this by moving a limiting past out of the way of the present and future which simplifies life) and continuation as well as figure-ground, this pattern points out the dangers of living in a past that can never truly be accessed again. Figure-ground, in this case, refers to time orientation—past, present or future.

Whatever a person places emphasis on becomes the figure while the rest makes up the past (ground). The pattern suggests that the listener make the present the figure while the past becomes the ground. The only useful time destination becomes one in the present that aims toward a target in the future. Identifying 'time' as a sort of flowing current that never stops, the listener receives motivation to exist in the present and develop a strategy that will lead her to a desired future.

As with all communication, the listener will try it on in her own life, as we explain with the concept of egocentricity. And, by considering how it fits now and in the future illustrates both inductive logic and generalization (I indicate how it fits throughout and especially with the line, 'rapidly coming back together then settling down to a smooth calm' (3rd paragraph.). The beneficial state resulting from a present and future orientation will subtly reinforce sustaining the time orientation through *transductive logic*, as it will create good outcomes resulting in continuation.

> This collection of letters band together to make words banded together to report an idea concerning your moving through time from the past to the future on a ship known as the *B Here Now*. You know you can choose your point of viewing your surroundings from any of 360 degrees. But do notice that the *B Here Now* only moves forward leaving the past behind. This ship can move forward slowly or quickly but move forward it does.
>
> You may observe from left to right and forward to behind, noticing the effect of the *B Here Now* moving forward through the water. And even if you decide to turn to the left or right you still move forward. If you decide to turn fully around, going back to where you came from, the *B Here Now* continues moving forward, not sideways or backwards. When you get back to where you left behind the water is forever changed, you know, stirred by your movement and trailing

wake. No way for the *B Here Now* to be there then again. This only delays progressing toward another desired destination.

Allow yourself to slowly shuffle back to the rear of the ship. Peer off the back noticing your *wake*. Notice the difference in the *wake* at the point closest to the ship, that most recently affected, and then how it changes, as you look further away. Also notice how the water parted by the *B Here Now* always reunites, rapidly coming back together then settling down to a smooth calm. It happens continuously, you know.

Looking further behind your ship, off in the distance, notice how all-visible traces of your past path vanish. By the way, who is choosing the direction and steering the *B Here Now*? Remember, your *wake* is past and the *B Here Now* continues moving. You may want to assert your preference for where. Otherwise, you'll be living in its *wake* and that does not propel the *B Here Now*, will it? In fact, it almost seems that a magnetic force exists pulling you toward whatever you decide to be your destination. Notice that setting a smooth course naturally follows fixing upon the destination you find the path leading you to where you want to go most.

Chapter Six
Section I: Language Patterns
Addressing Perception

Why do we utilize hypnotic patterns to address perception? Consider this. In order for you to experience a state of mind-emotion, you must have perceived some stimuli within yourself or from within your environment. Either stimulus, internal or external, will be consistent with the state it stimulated. If the state of mind-emotion is not consistent with the stimuli perceived we refer to that as dissonance. This refers to a jarring and disruption of consciousness. If we are in a state of joy and receive some mildly bad news, we experience dissonance. Either the bad news (stimulus) is deleted or the state shifts to be in accord with the bad news.

> **If the state of mind-emotion is not consistent with the stimuli perceived we refer to that as dissonance.**
>
> **Since people strive for dissonance reduction through consistency of state and perception, they will alter state or perception to eliminate the dissonance.**

Since people strive for dissonance reduction through consistency of state and perception, they will alter state or perception to eliminate the dissonance. A person can change his perception by changing the state of mind-emotion. Or, this person can change her state by changing what or how he perceives. It is the latter of these two methods that makes up the content of this next section.

Perceptions function as self-organizing systems. Perceptions act as 'attractors' in that they attract those things in the environment that support their existence. Beliefs notoriously do this. If I believe that the world is 'out to get me' than all I will see, hear and feel are those events that I interpret as 'out to get me'. Everything else will either be deleted out or distorted to fit my perception. Our perceptions become our filters through which we view and experience our world. This corresponds to the NLP model that states that our unconscious filters (language, memories, decisions, Meta-programs, beliefs, values and attitudes) serve to delete, distort and generalize all incoming and outgoing data.

When you have an experience of joy and you are in the outdoors, doesn't the air seem cleaner and fresher? During a state of joy colors often appear brighter; food tastes better and things even sound better. The birds sing louder and the music notes of your favorite tunes seem to touch you more. Physically you may experience an energized sensation or a feeling of lightness. You will more likely notice the good in all that exists around you while dismissing the bad. This perceptual pattern begets more joy thus fulfilling the Gestalt principle of continuation. In doing so you sustain the state induced by your perception. You perceive in patterns consistent with your state of mind-emotion unless otherwise shifted. If you shift perception, you will then perceive stimuli corresponding to the state.

States can shift as a result of perceiving different information in the environment. An example of how states and perception work hand in hand follows. Over your lifetime you have, no doubt, achieved many goals. If you have put a great deal of effort into achieving various goals, which you probably have done, no doubt there have been a few times that you did not attain your desired goals. These two sets of information can represent vastly different categories. Some people can reminisce about their accomplishments and find they associate into a positive, effective state of mind-emotion. A person in a very positive, effective state will be more likely to be aware of his successes. Another person may equate failure at attaining goals as indicative of failure as a person. Such a person will associate into a more negative state of mind-emotion.

The two factors, states and perceptions, work hand in hand to form a person's subjective reality. *When states and perceptions are at odds, dissonance exists.* And that's the jarring we feel on the inside. The relationship between states and perception also holds true with regard to limiting states and unsuccessful performances. A person could associate into a limiting state if focusing on just unsuccessful efforts. While in a limiting state, a person will most likely notice his own shortcomings.

It seems that when we perceive dissimilar stimuli for more than just a moment, we dismiss the initial differences due to our need to group for similarity and dissonance reduction. The perceiver may delete the dissimilar or distort the traits of the stimuli to create the illusion that they are similar. And if she cannot do that, the perceiver will tend to find a different category that fits the differing stimuli. The adjustments in perception necessary for grouping dissimilar stimuli into a larger, more inclusive category, often result in a shift in states of mind-emotion. The larger category is a Meta-category. After the state shift occurs the perceiving shift will take care of itself since the state determines what we perceive.

A case involving a married couple provides an example of categorizing stimuli and their effect on states. The wife described a pattern of arguing in which a disagreement would trigger memories of her previous unpleasant experiences with her husband (known as anchors in NLP). Once arguing about a single issue, she would only recall all the bad things that her husband had said and done to her. This 'all or nothing thinking' limited her awareness and responses along with restricting her state of mind-emotion. This limiting perception caused significant conflicts between the two.

Once this woman described how she created her great anger, I asked her a simple question that required a perceptual shift to answer. I asked, 'What would you feel instead of anger and how would you respond instead of yelling when you think about both your husband's good and bad behavior at the same time?' She immediately changed facial expressions. Her face became less tense. She stated that she would see him differently and that she would not feel so mad when he behaved in ways she did not like. This would result in her not yelling at him.

By recognizing his good side, she would also be more likely to talk out her concerns with him regarding just his behavior—keeping his personhood separate from his behavior. The husband certainly liked this concept and stated he believed he could be less defensive and more engaging in future discussions with her. With this perceptual shift, we then began to work on conflict resolution skills to address the specific conflict issues in the marriage. Before she resolved this issue, we could only talk about her global thought—'He is a bad person'.

> **These language patterns take advantage of the naturally occurring either–or dichotomy in human perception. You perceive either the figure or the ground from a whole stimulus. The figure becomes known in detail while the ground remains vague.**

So a change of state can result from directly addressing the state or accumulating sufficient counter evidence from altered perception to persuade a state shift. This latter path makes up the focus for the hypnotic patterns in this section. These language patterns take advantage of the naturally occurring either–or dichotomy in human perception. You perceive either the figure or the ground from a whole stimulus. The figure becomes known in detail while the ground remains vague. In general, the figure makes up primary awareness while ground comprises secondary awareness.

Since we often perceive in either–or ways, the content of the figure plays a crucial role in determining and sustaining state. By shifting what you perceive to the ground information, different information from the ground becomes known and integrated. This different information forces the client to alter her state because the stimuli differs and creates cognitive dissonance. The information and belief no longer match so the state finds no grounds to support the old belief.

> **Shifting from the old figure to the varied stimuli in the ground lets new possibilities come into awareness.**

Shifting from the old figure to the varied stimuli in the ground lets new possibilities come into awareness. This shifting of perception can occur about the significant event by triggering awareness of new information in the background. You may ask someone who nervously describes how she almost became involved in a car accident 'What did this almost accident, not do?' This provides an example of asking for awareness of information not initially noticed such as an absence of damage and presence of safety in this case. By asking, 'What is 'not' the problem?' you force the client's perception from what she has in conscious awareness (figure) to everything else (ground). And how do you feel now noticing this?

> **By asking, 'What is 'not' the problem?' you force the client's perception from what she has in conscious awareness (figure) to everything else (ground).**

You may also shift perception by first addressing the general perceptual style of the client by utilizing something unrelated to her problem. For instance, ask a person to notice all the blue colored items in a room for a 20-second period. Follow this by asking him to describe all the green items in that same room. Once accessing the ability to notice ground in a neutral situation, for example, you can then apply the new style like a template laid over the stimuli that made up the significant event. 'Just like you shifted from noticing blue to noticing green, what do you now notice about your situation that is different from what you first noticed'? NLP students will recognize that in effect you 'Swish' the 'figure to the ground' and the 'ground to the figure.'

The section that follows consists of hypnotic patterns that address general perception styles rather than specific issues. These can be used to shift client perception and then re-examine the specific issues facing the client. When applied to an existing problem this shift in perception allows new information and resourceful responses.

Air Hole: *Reversing Perceptual Figure-Ground*

The words in this pattern address specifically what NLP refers to as Meta-programs or perceptual filters. The purpose here is to take long-standing figure (conscious) assumptions and turn them inside out. This will result in providing a new perspective for the client as he accesses information in the ground (unconscious mind). Once this loosening occurs, the client can apply the new found information to a more specific issue within the therapeutic process.

> **Once perceptual filters loosen, the state becomes vulnerable and amenable to change.**

The foundation for this process consists of the gestalt concept of dissonance. The words presented below make for dissonance in existing perceptions by confusing the listener. Once perceptual filters loosen, the state becomes vulnerable and amenable to change. Toward the end of the pattern, a sort of 'time travel' occurs. The listener goes back to his original condition, where no holes or problems exist (the 'void', the 'place of pure potentiality' or 'before words'). From the original condition the client receives word that everything following the original condition is essentially artificial, human-made and superimposed and, therefore, totally changeable.

The purpose here is to remind the listener of his 'whole nature' (similarity with the use of hole-whole—a phonological ambiguity) and that this ultimately remains intact regardless of what happens to them in life. A double bind happens near the end when the listener is asked to 'go deeper, gradually or quickly'. Similarity occurs with the use of 'fore' for 'for'—a phonological ambiguity.

> Have you ever accidentally torn a hole in a piece of clothing, either while you were wearing it or while you were not? It can be upsetting, especially if the shirt, skirt, pants, coat or blouse is a favorite of yours. For some items you can get replacement cloth to fill in for the separated cloth. You call these patches. They span the gulf, covering the *hole*.
>
> You may tend to see the space between the once joined cloth as the material having a *hole* in it. But have you ever stopped to think that the material is actually causing a hole in the air. It sort of separates the once-joined air by placing the cloth in between.
>
> The cloth tearing may actually be the air returning to its original condition of just air without a tear. So which has the hole, the material or the air? It all depends on what you decide is

background and what is fore. Another way of looking at this dilemma is determining which came first, the air or the material. Did the material just spring out of thin air? Or did the air just spring out of thin material?

Now consider this consideration applying to any and all situations. Which is template and which is original, which came first? Look at each, and then decide so that your clear and full perceiving comes first and your decision is the template over the vast expanse of awareness preceding. Going deeper, gradually or quickly become aware that the you, you know, once were *whole* without any *holes*, complete. Know the original condition and work from there. Get a feel for the material. Anything that tears or is capable of tearing is just superimposed.

The Map is Some Territory: *Sorting for Differences*

Several perceptual styles receive attention here. Noticing similarities and over generalizing (referring to confusing street names), continuation, along with pointing out the 'not' or gap where similarities end and differences begin, make up the perceptual styles highlighted in this pattern. The word collection begins with a rather universal experience of noticing similar street names in different cities. This helps to address egocentricity. The different cities serve to represent different situations.

Drawing upon the uniqueness of each situational state, I address the state of 'comfort'. Comfort, as a state, tends to promote continuation because the person experiencing comfort often believes it is simpler to just stay comfortable. Finding cues to detect differences forms an essential influence in affecting desired outcomes in different circumstances. Calling on states of mind-emotion and remembering the infinite possibilities, which broadens awareness, are essential ingredients for successful outcomes. 'Calling on states of mind-emotion' occurs by referencing 'maps of states' and the reference to 'all roads existing and proposed'.

The pattern leads the listener through the 'lost' to the 'found' to the 'internal resources' he desires to use. Once again, the big three steps present in change show up here, associating into the problem, dissociating from the problem and associating into a resourceful state or perceptual mode.

As you think back on your various travels to different cities and states over the years, have you ever found different cities and states have streets with the same names? It immediately reminds you of home and then you notice how the streets compare in terms of what lines each side of them.

After you notice the general name similarity you then notice the differences—the gap. It always seems amazing to find a street with the same name on a different map, sort of like meeting a neighbor from home in a foreign country, rather comforting. Yet this perspective remains narrow, increasing the possibility of missing the bigger picture.

Not all nests are alike to the lookalike birds we know as the sparrow. No matter how careful the aim, no path is ever the same, even for the very next arrow. So how do you keep from getting thrown off course, and if you do just get right back on, by those times when you find major similarities tempting to evoke the same old response? It's not in the details. If you seek a street and know the name avoid seeking all the same. The list will boggle and push you from one end to the other and still you will not.

Instead, start with the state then open this map to find the path you seek. It starts with a certain state then moves to the city followed by more specific still, until you find the line by the name you want. To find a brown bear you don't start with all animals that are brown. You start with the bare facts then get down to brass tacks. So choose a state before you navigate your path. It will guide you to find any and all roads paved, unpaved and yet to be paved. You know, those different colored lines known as proposed. This of course depends on your need. So God speed you to the proper state then city then part of town then street then address then building inside to find exactly what you came for.

Whose Reality is it Anyway? *Identifying Personal Boundaries*

The content of this pattern asks the listener to determine what she holds as truth for herself. Any co-dependent type of behavior may benefit from this pattern. The language pattern describes the general dynamics of interacting with another person. The foundation of beliefs and values then comes into play. These latter two elements, beliefs and values, determine what a person holds as true. Therefore, accessing values and beliefs allows more clarity and a more effective screening device for deciding behavioral choices.

Noting the drawbacks and pitfalls of going too far by using all of someone else's reality or rigidly holding one's own, invokes secondary awareness. A person must access secondary awareness in order to process and consider the three reality points of: all yours, all mine, and somewhere in between. Knowing where to draw the line and why to draw the line permits more effective functioning.

> We each perceive our surroundings from unique perspectives. We each process this perception collection in unique ways making meaning as distinct as your DNA. You know how a strawberry tastes but cannot fully convey this to me. You can start the description but I have to taste the strawberry to make sense to myself.
>
> Experience is the best, if not only, teacher. Every time you interact with someone, part of the time spent together gets used determining and agreeing on what reality is to be used for this occasion. Some people find it easy to mutually agree on a reality for any event. Others seem to require you to use theirs. Not out of generosity but out of felt necessity. Theirs is organized in just such a way as to permit them comfort. For them to accommodate you means insecurity in their world, nothing personal, of course. In fact that sort of reality prevents anything personal from happening, insuring further insecurity.
>
> Now some people ask you use their reality and if your reality includes living within someone else's reality then you have a comfortable fit. This appears quite the opposite in word and deed from an anger fit. This occurs when realities rub but don't blend. The friction results in a reality quake along a fault line.

Notice where your reality is and is not, of course each is your reality. It's just some is considered out of bounds. Do you use your reality or does your reality call for you to use that of others? Usually you can feel when someone else asks you to live according to his or her reality. Doing so requires a degree of contorting on your part.

You also have to deny certain beliefs. If you do a very good job of this you deny you deny. Mission impossible, you know the show, disavow any knowledge of your past. Similar realities naturally band together it is the worlds way, birds of a feather. You choose your reality you choose your band. Name that tune before it begins.

Reversing the order of things ends you up waiting in a room full of waiters with no chef. So how do you decide what you will use to construct your reality and how do you do? Is reality yours, mine or ours? Just whose reality is it anyway?

Yes Yes Yes Yes Yes NO!! Limit Setting

This language pattern comments on one of Newton's laws of physics, which states that a body in motion tends to stay in motion. Most people tend to just continue patterns of habitual thinking, emotions and behaviors in a rather auto pilot way unless something clearly blocks their path. The continuation perceptual principle plays the crucial role in this pattern.

The pattern as a whole raises the issue of when and where to put a stop to a habitual thought, emotion or behavior. The intervention applied here suggests shifting the nominal level of data, all-or-nothing perspective, to a more sophisticated means of detecting and setting boundaries. The limit testing invites thinking outside the bounds and results in identifying categories by criteria.

The process within the language suggests that the listener recognizes the denominalized nature of 'nature'. Nothing in nature exists in a static form. 'Nature' continually ebbs and flows. Using the natural human tendency to find similar examples (similarity), the denominalized perspective on a specific behavior addressed with the hypnotic pattern will just naturally be applied to other facets of behaviors in other contexts. This foresight then receives encouragement for generalization. Dissonance, or confusion, takes place in the very first line with the word 'repeat' repeating itself. Meta-programs or perceptual filters receive attention as well by suggesting alternative points of view on old information. Figure and ground, in particular, get questioned at the end of the second paragraph.

> It can be sort of interesting to notice how patterns repeat repeat themselves. Once we get on a roll we tend to continue repeating the same response. Some people call them habits but you know the pattern. It's one of those innate human tendencies. Newton even decided it is a law of nature. A body at rest tends to stay at rest. But is anything ever completely still? Only if the temperature rests at absolute zero, -432 degrees.
>
> The other half of the equation is a body in motion tends to stay in motion. And what if you get a notion to rest on the motion of the ocean, driftwood, at the mercy of the current trends. When you shift from, to.... how do you know what changed? You know it's all in how you look at things and compare them. If a person gets laid off from his job he may say he is in-between jobs. But what if his job was in-between layoffs?
>
> Notice the difference the different view affords. Background becomes foreground and foreground becomes background. The rainy day is in-between sunny days or the sunny day is in-between rainy days. What is the reference point and how does it feel using the pleasant as the reference? Don't you find … you gravitate?
>
> Newton revisited. What is at rest and motion? If you can read five minutes than you can read six, right? And if you can read six minutes you can read seven. When do you put a stop to the progression so you will not end up reading in continual succession? And if you decrease what keeps you from permanently ceasing? What do you want to put in motion while the rest of you follows? And remember, just because it rests doesn't mean you can't give it a motion notion to come forward. Decide what you want to repeat and how will you k-n-o-w…if it works?

Lines: Removing Mental Structure to Allow Choice

Recognize that any linguistic structure can revert back, one step at a time, to become what it was before it was the structure it is.

The listener may return to the place of pure potentiality (the 'void', 'beyond or before words') during this pattern. Recognize that any linguistic structure can revert back, one step at a time, to become what it was before it was the structure it is. Recently, I used an example of a client's shoe to take her back to the place that contains all and nothing at the same time. The shoe was noted as coming from her collection at home. But that came from the larger store collection—from the larger warehouse collection—from the larger manufacturer—from the designer of all to the raw materials —to cotton plants (she wore cotton upper sneakers)—to before the first cotton plant and what is there, anything and everything yet to be. The process proved effective for the client.

The current pattern describes the four lines used in forming a square. The listener is asked to visualize a square and then gradually alter the square until it vanishes. The words then tell the listener that all opportunities for resources and shapes reside within the self and are available to her. Following this awareness, the listener gets invited to continue and to apply these resources wherever and however she desires.

By identifying four factors that shape states of mind, thought, emotion, sensation and behavior in the first sentence, the pattern evolves by inviting the client to process complex data (interval and ratio) and higher-level thinking. Now that the pattern has activated complex thought capacity to more abstract symbolic figures, we have gained entry into the ground or secondary awareness.

> While you may act a certain way at this time, you may think of this current way as being a collection of thoughts, emotions, sensations and behaviors, four parts. You may also think of this current way as being like the four lines of equal length connecting to make a square. And this square actually includes some things and excludes some things just by its closed nature.

These four lines of equal length can alter some by having the two vertical or upright lines lean to the left or right, to some degree, while still connected at the four corners. Now you have what is called a parallelogram, is that two telegrams sent side by side [*dissonance-confusion producing*]?

If the two upright lines slant more you still have a parallelogram but if they slant so much they all become horizontal then you just have four straight lines overlapping each other becoming one setting free the contents. The lines contain nothing then, do they? And you can just send these four lines away clearing your drawing screen.

Yet you can remember the four lines in any form from straight line to square, knowing it remains in storage along with all the infinite number of lines and shapes you contain containing various resources yet to be in any form so you may choose to choose for the shape of things you want around you knowing you store all lines and shapes with the possibility of creating any design you desire, now don't you?

Status Quo Foe: Noticing Options for Change

Awareness of choice, figure-ground, dissonance and similarity primarily comprise this pattern. Similarity occurs with the use of the phrase 'allows one to…or more' (3rd paragraph) and 'a hat that goes on ahead' (next to last paragraph). Dissonance occurs with the pattern as a whole as previous states or beliefs get challenged and replaced with a different idea. The different idea requires the listener to reconcile the old with the new.

The figure-ground interplay occurs with referring to the 'fleet of all cars existing' (2nd paragraph) and by the thought of selecting a tape different from the one now playing. The purpose here is to increase the awareness of what the listener is not doing or noticing. This accenting the 'not' points the listener to his unconscious mind. Options, options and more options occur through this piece serving to remind the listener of overall choice.

The listener receives a request to search the past when the second sentence of the first paragraph asks, 'How much sooner it could have been what is now.' This works with past awareness of the unconscious mind. The sentence structure notes the cues from previous learning about the timing of change. Very often a person will delay making change even when the situation and time for change are right. So here, the listener gets asked to compare, think about and utilize past learnings in the present.

In the next to last paragraph referring to the 'hat that goes on ahead' and then proceeding into the future makes for confusion or dissonance as well as using similarity. The sentence following the confusion point is the one with a significant opportunity to influence thoughts, emotions and behavior. So presenting the desired outcome here can help make it happen.

The pattern invites secondary awareness with the reference to the opposite sorting style of the tape player seeking silence rather than sound. This refers to the 'not' or unconscious mind. In this case, the 'not' comprises the ground and the conscious mind comprises the figure. Different levels of change present themselves through referring to changing tunes or changing whole tapes. The 'fleet of all cars existing' in the second paragraph, suggests all possibilities in the pool of choices. Several similarities of both sound and meaning, tune ahead, occur in this pattern.

> Some things change or evolve over time. After they become different or modified you may wonder how much sooner it could have been what it is now. With this in mind consider the music systems that come in cars, vans and vehicles in general. Originally, no radio existed in the early vehicles and later just a radio and speaker. Then the radio added a tape player and more speakers. Now the tape player is more sophisticated along with the additional speakers.

> And if your car was not one of the early ones to have some of these features you might first find out when you had occasion to rent a car while traveling for business or fun. You may experience renting a car from the fleet of all cars existing and find a cassette tape left by the previous renter, much to all's surprise. And you can place the cassette in the tape player because you're naturally curious to play this unknown music. You wait eagerly with open mind and ears.

> The tape player is the kind that allows one to...or more searches for just the right tune if the current one is

dissatisfying. Simply push the button and the tape player somehow knows to search for the silence between tunes instead of the usual attending to sound. It seeks not sound but is based on sound principles you know because it works well.

If the tune playing is not satisfying simply push the search button and the tape player will shift to the next tune for your listening to determine if you like it more. It only stays the same when we forget it can be different. Wondering about different possibilities…is the way to making different. What is amenable? Whatever you believe.

I once knew someone who believed your past does not affect your present or future. I wonder when in his past he chose that belief and how does it not affect his present and future? If you do not find the tune playing satisfying, simply push the button again and search for the next selection on the tape. Some mechanism within acts like a hat that goes on ahead …. looking for what is desired and what will it do when it gets there knowing…that it already knows … how to cause what it wants consistent with its cause … because, it is one with you.

If the entire tape seems dissatisfying just remove it and replace it with one consistent with your wants to be satisfied and you know this feeling now … only propels you forward in a similar detecting manner as the tape player, only seeking what satisfies consistent with purpose knowing exactly what this is and really always has been, is and will be, won't it?

Why Not: Getting Beyond the Why Question

The words contained below simply address the tendency for some people to need to know 'why' everything happens. This tendency interferes with the therapeutic process as often the 'why' person can't suspend his 'why' investigative nature enough to actually experience the process and then find out why. The 'why' person frequently wants to analyze before the therapy takes place rather than afterwards. This type of person embodies the theory that the conscious mind surely knows how to get in the way of unconscious change. On many occasions I precede an intervention with a 'why' person with this pattern or some excerpt from it.

If more dissonance seems called for, I will utilize the whole pattern or some spin-off from it. If the person has a less than overwhelming 'why' within them, I'll just ask the question, 'When you have what you want, will you care why you didn't?' I've found this preamble effective every time I apply it. The question shifts the listener to the outcome rather than focusing them on the processes of the therapy. The question invites the person to leave the present and to imagine her future outcome as already happening.

The extended pattern also utilizes humor ('a why knot') along with a reframing of the purpose of the 'why'. This allows a more effective use of this actual solution search strategy. I believe this reframing simplifies the 'why' process and leads the person to keep the 'why' after, rather than before, the change process. Thus the interruptive conscious mind takes a back seat until the change occurs. The extended pattern also employs similarity in the fifth line with 'be...cause...instead' to both address the 'why' question with 'because' and invites the listener to take a proactive role choosing to be at 'cause' (choice) rather than at 'effect' in her life.

> For those of you who feel a need to know why for all things, this is for you. Of course you now wonder *why* but let's not delay. Keeping with the inevitable parallel process, I now wonder *why* you need to know *why* and what would happen if you applied your need to know *why* to your need to know *why* (a Meta-stating process). I imagine you would tie yourself up in *a why knot* for ages.

> And just *why* do you need to know *why* ... be ... cause ... instead ... when you have what you did not have or feel how you did not feel will you care *why* not? Perhaps your need to know *why* only wants security because knowing *why* will allow awareness of the foundation so you can repeat the performance. And I wonder if your need to know *why* would do better if it focused on how, to keep and use what you got instead of *why* you got it because spending time on *why* only delays enjoying what. Now you've got it.

Comparisons: *Getting Beyond Either–Or Thinking*

The content of this word collection addresses the process used when comparing any two or more items. The original act of comparing seems to stem from noting similarities but eventually leads to noticing differences as well. The purpose of this pattern is to highlight both the similarities and the differences. By highlighting both similarities and differences, we eliminate the either–or perspective that limits awareness and choice.

Figure-ground relations, involving similarities–differences, serve as the prime target with continuation encouraged. In this sense, figure serves as the content of the conscious mind while ground makes up the unconscious mind. Thus the 'similarities' invoke the 'conscious mind' or figure; and 'differences' invoke the 'unconscious mind' or ground.

By not addressing the future, the drive for closure will lead the client to fill in the missing piece, thus the client will, hopefully, automatically future pace themselves. By not addressing the future, this works as an Ericksonian 'incomplete sentence' or continuation as the client unconsciously fills in what is missing. The pattern itself becomes an example of its own point by leading the client to first notice compatible pieces and then to see the differences. The awareness of differences utilizes the 'not' primary awareness, which leads the client directly to her secondary awareness where she can access her pool of unconscious resources.

> You can look back in your past and know that when you notice something the noticing results from initially comparing so you can decide what to notice. And yet, when you compare two items in the world around you, saying one is like the other, you also automatically notice how they are not alike, don't you? And this you may like, more than how they are alike. In fact you can make differences declare themselves by stating two items are alike. The differences will announce themselves clearly and strongly. This uncovering may assist in identifying more useful information or resources you can use now.

The Ladder of the Two: *Accessing Meta-States through Perceptual Shifts*

This pattern utilizes a person's ability to shift perspectives and access higher and broader points of view. The foundation for climbing to these higher perspectives comes in a time reference that disorients the client and creates dissonance. The listener is invited to consider past, present and future, which will dissociate the person from the present state, permitting access to higher states. Also, invoking multiple senses ('saw, felt or heard') provides a deeper immersion into the trance. Think of each 'sense invoked' as a weight on a diver at sea. With each sense, or weight, the diver just goes deeper.

Once reaching a higher perspective within the metaphor, the listener gets invited to dissociate. Dissociating sends the client Meta to his higher perspective. This allows a change in perception of both self and environment. Additionally, the listener receives reinforcement for his sense of 'internal knowing' through use of dissociation and similarity with the phrase 'you know'.

The metaphor of climbing a ladder serves to provide the means by which the client achieves higher and broader perceptions. Considerable dissonance, similarity and continuation come into play. The dissonance takes place with the initial time references and noting the points of view of others. The use of 'ring' and 'wrung' bring similarity principles into play. Repeated use of the phrase 'you know' brings further dissonance and dissociating out of past limitations into a position of choice. While the early portion of this pattern involves time reference, the pattern ultimately aims at altering perception.

> As you tune into your self and your parts within you, you can become aware of different perspectives about past, present or future issues. You know you saw or felt or heard things from others' perspectives and then your own. Remembering your past you know this rings true. It always rings unlike the ladder with rungs. It always rung just waiting for you to answer and step to a rung answering the call to step up higher and see what you can see from an elevated perspective. And you know it contains more rungs for you to step up to seeing even more … broader and deeper views.

And while you place yourself up on as high a rung as you like you can also notice that you know you reside here. This is interesting because where is the you that knows you know you stand there, you know? And now notice the perspective that you get from noticing you standing on as high a rung as you like, being aware of what you know from up there about what goes on below you. So now you know you know you know that you know how to use this now and how from here on, see?

Figure and Ground: Finding Your Significance as a Person

While this hypnotic pattern may seem obvious as to the issue it addresses, it also strives to use this figure-ground arrangement to initiate an unconscious state change. This pattern seeks to identify with that individual who struggles with feelings of insignificance. The pattern first associates the person into the problem state of 'insignificance' and then moves them out of it.

Early in this pattern the listener is invited to step into an awareness of the existing 'wonders of the world'. To do this, the person tunes into observing great natural structures with reference to the possibility of more than just 'seven wonders of the world' existing. The pattern directs the client's attention to the 'seventh heaven' (a familiar term to many in the religious world) to gain a more pleasant resourceful Meta-state. Hopefully, by now, the client has dissociated from their problem state of feelings of insignificance (figure) and has associated into a more resourceful Meta-State (ground).

Now you can convey the real message. The listener receives a message of hope and of universal interacting as she experiences alternating roles of support. At the same time, the client finds herself achieving the spotlight role, which eliminates the feelings of insignificance. Everyone contributes to the greater good.

The ultimate target of this pattern is reassuring the listener that she possesses value and has much to offer others and the universe in a meaningful way. Impetus for continuing this pattern of thought is given at the end in the form of double meaning (similarity or phonological ambiguity) with the word 'vital' suggesting that the listener first steps into the state of feeling 'vital'. This invites a feeling of being a 'vital' part of the world, which, hopefully, will motivate the listener to continue in this state and role.

The first paragraph serves as a preamble in assisting the client in understanding and setting the frame for the pattern. It will be a helpful sort of introduction to the pattern.

> In order for you to question or doubt your worth you have to have a particular focus. And you have to have some other information out of focus. What you focus on is called the figure, since it is the figure of your attention. What you ignore and do not focus on is called the ground. This ground is sort of like a background. And if you do a background check you may then find vital information that is useful to you now.
>
> And if you ever wonder, and by the way, you know there are seven wonders of the world, and I suppose you can wonder more as you like. But the number seven is interesting and seems to symbolize high points such as the seventh heaven being the best one. Now keeping this in mind please be aware that we each play either the number seven or make up all the other numbers without which the number seven would have no significance.
>
> As people we are all either figure or ground. You cannot be neither, go figure. The flower rising up from its root in the soil could not be if it were not for the soil. We sometimes seem to forget the role of the soil but good gardeners remember to amend and toil so the soil will assist the flower in growing to full bloom for all to enjoy. In fact if it were not for the soil being just so there would be no flower bloom to enjoy. Such numerous colors and variety. And you know there is even sevin dust [*Sevin Dust—an insecticide used heavily in the US*] to help the process. The two parts, soil and flower, remain inseparable. In fact if they are separated each becomes a void.
>
> Now moving this figure-ground notion to the ocean, sometimes we take the role of the wave and sometimes we ride the surfboard. But I doubt the surf is bored. [*With this line about the 'surf' and 'bored,' what image comes to your mind and what does a person use this for in the tangible world?*] We all make waves or ride the crest of the waves but none of us are not wet. You may not make big waves but you contribute with all

the wave makers and together provide the impetus and support upon which others glide and stand out. In some sense the surfer can only do what us wave makers allow. You are cause and effect the surfer.

At various times and in various settings you invariably play each, foreground and background. Nobody is just background. You are each fore at some points as well. Nobody goes without contributing regardless of which role she plays. There exists flower or soil, surf or surfer and the displays go well beyond seven. For more, consider the racetrack and the horse, the air and the airplane, the canvas and the painting, the field and the game, the movie star is not this without certain behavior by those not on camera, your learning, planning and your harvest, notice and welcome it all knowing the real cause and effect is vital.

Go Off: *Bringing Conscious Choice to Habitual Responses*

The goal in this pattern involves the figure-ground play by loosening up the meanings associated with certain common phrases. Playing with these phrases makes use of similarity or phonological ambiguity. This loosens the grip of primary awareness that tends to lock in only one meaning. After loosening up primary awareness, one can then activate secondary awareness.

Drawing on the auditory and visual sense allows for a fuller experience for the listener. I imply continuation because once a process starts in motion, it tends to continue in motion. Continuation receives a 'not too subtle shove' with the last sentence. Invoking the state of curiosity towards the end invokes a useful resource for propelling the figure-ground perceptual shift into the future. This happens as the client wonders where and how this 'strange' language applies.

> You know some words or phrases may sound the same but they have completely opposite meanings. I mean, consider the short phrase '*go off*'. When you make the television *go off* it becomes totally silent and blank without a picture. But when you make a rocket *go off* it becomes extremely loud and very bright, not to mention moving.

Now consider the phrase *'go on'*. When you say it one time you may mean that you want a person to stop what she is doing and leave. But when the same person says or does something interesting that grabs your curiosity, pulling you closer, you tell her to *go on* because you want her to continue. So now you can decide what you want to *go off* and what you want to *go on* in you, and how you intend it, can't you?

Locking In: Setting Boundary Lines

Figure-ground along with boundaries receive attention here. The beginning part of the script invites the listener to go into trance by narrowing the focus of awareness and then generating flexibility by shifting the focus. This leads to a more useful focus by applying awareness to boundary lines in relationships or other life tasks. The pattern permits the unconscious mind to determine where to draw the boundary lines that conform to the listener's purpose. This design attempts to highlight the thought process involved in deciding what to include and exclude when drawing boundary lines.

Addressing the need for safety underlines the pattern in general. Why else do we draw the lines where we do but, ultimately, for safety? Yes, the line is drawn where it is because it works this way. But why is it not drawn elsewhere? Because it would not work elsewhere which would end up endangering the person. The absence of boundaries quickly becomes overwhelming and unmanageable leading to unsafe conditions. This invokes cognitive dissonance, which directs the client in drawing safe boundaries.

> Drawing on your past experience, you know, you can apply your energy focus to any specific area like a free-floating magnifying glass that hovers or lands anywhere needing a closer look. For example you do this when you focus your attention on your left big toe. You do this when you focus your attention on your right index finger or the top of your head off which many good ideas come.
>
> Oddly, this top of the head notion, that the thought emerges without much in depth thinking, is a misnomer. These off the top ideas stem from your deepest roots you feel all the way

down in you. Your unconscious mind simply uses the elevator to the top floor. It's an elevator not a dumbwaiter—it's just dumb to wait when you know your deepest unconscious sends you a thought requiring no thought on your conscious part.

Trust holds the key for unlocking the door. It's a skeleton key. You know the kind fitting all doors allowing choice emerging. Fear is the dead-bolt locking choice in for supposed safekeeping. But you can't spend any of the money while locked in the vault. Now notice that if something is locked in then something else is locked out. Which part do you focus on?

How can you rise above, focusing on both parts at once and even notice the third part, the dividing line? For a moment just shift your focus back and forth from the in to the out. Do this several times for note taking. Now we do need categories and these dividing lines allow this but these lines are movable. Notice you can set the line wherever best fits your want, locking in, locking out, or, perhaps, just making permanently permeable, your choice.

Map Reading: *Matching Choice to Current Contexts*

These words serve as a metaphor for the process a person uses in deciding what to do or how to accomplish an outcome. We tend to rely first on old information. But this old information may be outdated which will lead to ineffective outcomes. The pattern below invites shifting awareness from primary —old map—to secondary awareness—new or yet to be created maps of life.

The gestalt principles of figure-ground (old map versus new map), simplicity (using up-to-date information simplifies reaching goals) and continuation play primary cognitive roles in giving this pattern its effectiveness. After using this pattern, it may be useful to follow up by asking the listener to consider a specific issue on which she is working. After considering a specific issue, ask the listener how she may now notice alternative paths towards finding solutions for this issue.

It can be difficult deciding which direction to go, sort of like looking at a map of some new territory and trying to figure out how to get somewhere. You know maps have been around just about ever since people started leaving from one place to go to another. Map making is supposed to result in a more helpful guide for those who travel. But so much changes over time that the date on the map really becomes very important because the date the map was made tells you how current the information is in it.

Maybe the first thing to do before using any map is to find out when it was made. Otherwise you may be going on incorrect information. Then you could hunt a path that you saw on the map forever and never find it because it may be gone or some new and easier path may exist now and you did not know. You know how change results in some things going away and other new things coming into existence.

So it is very important to notice the newness of the map as you unfurl it, opening it up to show all the paths and desti-nations as you look north and south, west and east and even beyond the map or in between roads where just space exists, imagining how it may be. What roads are gone in favor of newer more convenient direct paths to where you want to go?

And even as you look at your newest map you can know that new paths are being created for you to travel on just as the ones existing now were once just planned. Notice how plan-ning leads to creation. And what do you want to plan to create now making a new road taking you to the outcome you most want now, aren't you?

Ballast: Raising the Level of Consciousness

The metaphor presented here represents ways a person attempts to reach higher levels of functioning. Sometimes a person attempts to sort of 'puff up' his ego and push himself to higher levels. This usually doesn't work because these efforts most often come from surface structure (conscious—figure) attempts rather than actu-ally altering internal personal contents (unconscious—ground).

The analogy of a hot air balloon provides the parallel process (isomorphism). The sandbags represent one's baggage or states of mind-emotion that serve to limit or to stop a person's progress. A direct correlation (isomorphic) exists between how many sand-bags a person carries and the need for 'over inflating' his balloon. The more bags released, the less need for hot air. The purpose of this pattern is to invite the listener to release his excess baggage. By releasing the excess baggage, the client may now naturally rise to higher levels of functioning.

Metaphors rely on the principle of egocentrism since the listener will always attempt to apply the message to self. Metaphors also rest upon a foundation of the gestalt principle of continuation. Once grasped, the listener will naturally continue applying and displaying the principle. Additionally, metaphors request the person to dissociate from his current perspective in order to associate into the perspective described within the metaphor. Metaphors resemble a ball thrown in the air. To catch it you must go where it is. Once there, you find a new perspective from this position. Essentially, a metaphor provides a symbolic reframe as opposed to the more literal application in reframing.

A person will always give, at least, a listen to a metaphor to determine if it holds merit in his life. The catchier the words used in describing the metaphor, the more likely the listener will try it on for himself thus yielding the desired results. In the case of hypnotic language, catchy words exemplify the gestalt principles noted earlier in the text and then just rely on the natural Piagetian cognitive processes to perform the task. The person listening will automatically organize what he hears by using figure-ground, simplicity, similarity, closure and continuation. The listener will also follow the cognitive 'rules' identified by Piaget by utilizing the principle conveyed within the metaphor.

> This story takes place in the early morning on a crystal clear day. You know the kind of day when the sky is so blue that you can look up at it and sort of see through it as far as you can imagine. It seems to have both substance and yet be permeable, you know, you can just go right through it. Well, on this early crystal clear morning a hot air balloonist and her balloon are ready for launch, launch not lunch. It is too early for lunch and timing is crucial you know. So this balloonist and her balloon prepare for launch. Her balloon is a wonderful shade of light blue. Such a shade that she can almost fade into the sky once up there.

Now that the device heating the air to fill the balloon is turned on, the balloon begins filling with hot air. The sort of folded blue sheet begins coming to life and taking shape, like a soldier coming to attention. Now ballooning, like most processes in life has two positions or directions available. You know the balloon must be able to go up but must also be able to come down. And for modifying the height sandbags are used.

Think about the beginner balloonist, this person may attach as many sandbags as possible out of fear to limit the height and the fear. Now the person with some experience may attach just enough sandbags that allow useful variation in altitude. This combined with the amount of hot air filling the balloon determines the height. However, the truly experienced expert balloonist may only use the sandbags to keep the balloon on the ground between uses.

Once deciding to inflate the balloon in order to rise, the sandbags are released one by one. As soon as the first sandbag drops away, the balloon begins rising. With each sandbag released, the balloon rises higher affording a new broader view, and you can see this can't you? You can almost see and then be the balloonist who decides to release the sandbags holding you down. Just flipping them over the side and watching them drop to the ground while you rise higher above it.

Notice how much smaller things look from up here. Everything is relative in size but it all looks smaller and smaller as you turn loose another sandbag. Feel the freedom surge lift you higher floating above all that rests below. How free does this feel and what else do you feel knowing you determine the height of your ascent? Rise as high as you like, simply release the sandbags. You can continue enjoying floating up on high as you know you independently control your altitude. [*Pause here for a moment to allow new awareness. You can also embellish with more and specifics here about some particular issue the client may have.*]

And you know when you want to come back to earth, remembering what you see and know… you can… just temporarily stop filling the balloon and gradually let the hot air out of the balloon, letting it slowly return you to earth while keeping the new height of knowing you now possess and feel, how it feels different. And be secure to remember you possess continual access to the device that inflates for lift-off any time you choose just inflate and release any and all sandbags. See how well it works for you to see how well it works?

Dilating: Expanding Awareness from Detail to Big Picture

This pattern aims to increase awareness by inviting the listener to shift from a narrow, foveal awareness, to a broader peripheral awareness. This also results in shifting from primary (foveal, focus) to secondary awareness (peripheral), thus accessing the resourcefulness of the unconscious mind. The gestalt principles and dynamics of simplicity, figure-ground (shifting from single focus to broad focus), similarity (lens-lends—a phonological ambiguity) and continuation apply in this pattern.

The shift of focus moves from narrow figure to broader ground, dissociating the person, and then returns to the narrow focus using a new perspective. The nearly ever-present cognitive principles of egocentricity and continuation also play a role in helping the words and suggestions within the pattern receive application to the listener's life.

Once you state this hypnotic pattern to a person, the listener's perception will shift from a narrow perspective to broad perspective. At this point, ask the listener to re-examine his concerns while retaining the broad awareness. Ask him what new information or ideas spring to mind with the new, more panoramic perspective.

> Well I know that you certainly see this situation in a particular way [*you, as the therapist, can specify just how the listener interprets the particular situation that he is dealing with*] and that you are sure of your take on this. You seem to have locked in on this particular interpretation of the circumstances, like ice encases a bud on a tree. Maybe you have seen photos of this spring event where the ice actually surrounds the bud. But what happens when the ice gradually melts allowing you to see what happens beyond the moment and the bud unfolds beyond what it is, into more than a bud, a flower or perhaps it is a fruit tree that bears fruit.

And what would it be like to take a photo of this? But would you use a zoom lens to see just the one or might you use a wide angle lens to notice all the blooms on this and the other trees allowing you to compare one bloom to another noticing how each is unique. And you can notice and know this, can't you, when you use your wide angle lens, it lends itself to an ever-broader view to help you view the new countless subtle variations as you look across, comparing.

And as you begin to see how each is different by scanning broadly and deeply to notice just how many differences exist, appreciating the uniqueness. Now notice how unique your own situation is and how you can see it and respond to it for what it is, unique. And just how do you want to use and respond to this unique situation to make it into what you most want, now for your future?

Look Where You're Going: Making Choices with Current Information

The words below address the tendency for people to rely on the past for behavioral choices in the present. Such behavior often results in repeating the past in the present and in the future regardless of whether or not it serves the person. Continuation plays a significant role in creating problems because a state or behavior continues in use beyond its usefulness. Knowing when to stop one style or strategy and start a different one marks successful people.

The idea behind this hypnotic pattern is to access the current strategy and then shift the listener away from it and into awareness of choice. Awareness of choice simplifies things. A person experiences freedom to choose the most appropriate strategy or state for any given situation, eliminating the complications created by old, self-limiting choices.

This particular hypnotic word collection first accesses the process of hindsight that must occur to perpetuate the past. After associating the listener into this process, the dissociating and shifting to the unconscious mind takes place. This shifting happens through dissonance (second paragraph and early third) and plays upon naturally occurring egocentricity as well as similarity by using the concept of rear view mirror. 'What a wreck' (similarity) invokes essential away-from strategies for preventing bad outcomes in the listener's life and further motivating a future orientation.

Now this may seem obvious but how do you navigate your course in front of you? You have to look where you are going of course. Yet we all seem to so often find ourselves repeating the same old behaviors regardless of how well it fits the situation.

How do you maintain the same old behavior time after time? Well hindsight is the crucial ingredient there. When faced with a situation in the present, the only way we can repeat the same response as used in the past is to look in the past through hindsight, a rearview mirror of sorts. You know, those backward looking lenses that seem to curve your vision from the present back around to our past. No matter how intensely you focus on the present, looking through the hindsight lens moves your vision to images of the past. You see how you responded then to a particular cue and like a good actor you find the same cue in the present, no matter how small or trivial, and take it as an action cue.

Do you ever ask how the scene went and if you'd like to do take two? What about rewriting the script to create a different ending sending the old script to the recycle bin for another time and place? Then using the familiar present cue to pivot off in a different direction, any one of the 359 will lead to a difference that can make a difference.

And if you wonder about the wisdom of this blindfolding your hindsight, consider the following, which of course requires activating your sight, fore and present. By the way, we know hindsight existed and you have foresight but what is clear sight of the present called? In another sense maybe it is nearsighted. This is external while insight is naturally internal, you sort of feel you know.

Returning to the wisdom of not relying on hindsight for present decisions, what will happen when you use hindsight for directing your driving on the road? Notice how you would have to look in the rearview mirror. What will happen when you go forward while looking backward? How long will that last? What a wreck! But of course you know the solution. And how is it that you know the solution, nearsight and foresight, now isn't this so . . . you can see where you are now and where you want to be? How clear!

Cactus Spotting: Identifying Desired Resources

The purpose of this language pattern is to shift the listener's awareness from one subject-object to another of a more useful nature —a figure-ground shift. The content is essentially a description of how to choose what you selectively attend to in the environment or in one's self. The language in the pattern promotes a dissociated perspective for the listener.

Each of us selectively attends stimuli on a continual basis. Deciding what best serves our purpose and then attending to it makes for more effective living. If you want to assist your client in finding and using state-behaviors such as assertiveness, sociability or some other state-behavior, this pattern can set the framework for identifying, tuning in and keeping the state-behavior. Once shifted, the continuation principle will naturally assist the listener in keeping this perspective for his benefit.

The description of events within the pattern provides instructions for how the listener can decide what to target for his focus and how to go about finding other examples of the resource. By resource I mean a behavior or a state of mind-emotion that may provide the necessary ingredients for solving an issue.

Using a general example of selective attending in the hypnotic pattern, the speaker can add at the end some specific resource or state as the target for the listener to find and then continue finding in the future. Perhaps you are helping your client become more assertive and the client has difficulty finding his assertive part of self. You can speak the pattern, providing the client with the general mindset of how to identify and continue identifying a desired target. You can then become more specific, asking the client to identify, find and apply assertiveness. This process can just as easily apply to states such as determination, motivation or any resource the client needs for a solution.

This hypnotic language set relies on similarity, simplicity, figure-ground and continuation for its effectiveness. The figure-ground interplay occurs with the searching for cacti while all other vegetation remains a blurred background. Acknowledging the relatively smaller stature of the cactus relates to the sought after personal resource of the listener. That resource lays sort of 'over-looked' and in the background of the listener's self.

The use of the phrase grown-up (similarity) invites a more mature perspective on the environment rather than a child-like perspective. The general setting of being at the coast and enjoying the sea breeze from a deck sets an atmosphere of a 'relaxed internal searching' from a dissociated state, thus decreasing defensiveness. Again, simplicity and continuation play a role in each pattern as Meta-stating simplifies any process and a person naturally continues applying material he just discovered.

> Not long ago while I was on vacation, I went to the East Coast and spent several days there. Now the location was up near the North Carolina–Virginia border. This area is not like the coast of South Carolina where palm trees grow. This area has different vegetation. There were even cacti growing there, cacti, you know, when there is more than one cactus. But these cacti grew quite small, about the size of a small house plant so they were hard to spot amongst all the other plants growing there that were mostly bigger.
>
> One day, before we actually noticed that there were cacti growing there, we were sitting out on the deck off the second floor of the house we rented. We just sat there enjoying the sea breeze and the view from the second floor.
>
> Suddenly someone noticed a cactus growing in the backyard of this house. It was just right there in the rather grown up yard. It took a moment for me to actually find the cactus within the grown up yard because it sort of blended in, being green and all. So I set my scan on cactus, you know, got the picture of a cactus in my mind and looked for those fan blade-like arms and the spikes coming out of those arms. Sure enough, from the observation deck, I finally spotted a cactus. I looked at it in some detail. It was really quite small and if I had not known what I was looking for I probably would not have noticed unless I stepped on it.

Now that I saw this cactus and took in the details of the size and shape, I began scanning the yard from my observation point. Sure enough, once I had my target, I began noticing more and more of these cacti. Every few feet I saw another right there within the grass. It was almost like these cacti were all I saw and everything else was just a blur that made up the background. I ignored everything else in finding these cacti. It became quite easy and I was amazed at just how many I spotted. They seemed everywhere.

And you can now decide what you want to find and spot it while all others that differ simply fade into the background making your cactus come forward into sharp focus for you to see.

Looking Left Turning Right: Detecting Essential Cues in the Environment

In this pattern I seek to lead the client to utilize several input sources in decision-making rather than forming a premature conclusion from just one information source. Some examples of similarity are present with my using the common phrases of 'right turn' and 'signals'. Also, I utilize the client's secondary awareness to override the tendency towards simplicity. Dissonance results from the multiple details presented in the story. By invoking dissonance, the listener will unconsciously access his secondary awareness in an attempt to process the details of the metaphor.

In *The User's Manual for the Brain* (1999), Michael Hall and I (BB) explain:

The basic component that drives the power of story or metaphor to transform meaning and change the formula arises from the story sharing a similar structure to our life and experiences. We call this similarity of structure, an isomorphic structure.

In a broader sense this story parallels (isomorphism) the general cognitive process of our accessing our own personal resources and then effectively and safely applying these resources to our life— making a safe right turn.

The goal of this pattern is to expand the listener's awareness so the listener can make more effective use and application of his own resources. Before stating this pattern, the presenter needs to be sure that the listener has a particular goal in mind and has access to specific resources that he will need to accomplish this goal. Stating this pattern after the listener identifies resources and a goal will naturally result in the listener applying the isomorphic words to the just elicited circumstance. The need to apply the words of the pattern to the most recently considered subject or object exemplifies the principles of simplicity, egocentrism and transductive logic.

> The other day a friend of mine was driving from the store to his home. He left the parking lot of the store where he went to get some much needed supplies. The way for him to get home was to turn right out of the parking lot. Naturally, before he turned right out of the parking lot he looked to his left to make sure it was clear. Now looking to his left he saw two lanes of traffic coming in his direction. Of course two lanes also go the other direction as well. About 50 yards to his left stood a traffic light which would help the turn happen when it turns red making the cars coming toward him have to stop for the light. This would leave an opening for him to turn. So he looked for cars coming in those two lanes and also he looked for cues to determine if they were slowing down for the changing traffic light.
>
> One particular car approaching in the left lane of the two lanes begins to slow down. So he began to wonder, really wanting to make sure, if it was now safe to turn. He could have used this as his only clue and just turned right out of the parking lot. But, he decided to look at another car coming in the right lane of the two lanes that was just a little behind the car in the left lane. He noticed this car was not slowing down yet so he looked back at the other car in the left lane of the two lanes and noticed the car now had on its turn signal to turn left and this was why it slowed down. A rather complicated set of signals and cues involved in just turning right but noticing them and interpreting them accurately really helps make your right turn, turn out right.

Section II
Language Patterns Addressing States and Behaviors Through Perceptual Shifts

The hypnotic language patterns in this section relate to more specific states or behaviors. The leverage for shifting of these states or behaviors comes from changing perception so as to prepare the client in becoming receptive to new information. This then encourages a shift in state or behavior to create more resourceful outcomes.

Play the Percentages: Pain Reduction

In the following hypnotic language pattern I address perception in two ways. First, the patterns revolve around either specific perceptual dynamics making up various issues or; second, they address general perceptual styles that can apply to a broad range of issues.

This pattern popped into my head while I was jogging around my neighborhood. At the time I did not know for whom or when the pattern would apply but I allowed it to unfurl. Later I found out just the right person for this pattern. The figure-ground interplay and its influence play a crucial role in this pattern. While the specific point of the words relates to pain reduction, the principle of reversing figure-ground may apply generally to any unwanted perception about self, others or life. The principle of the pattern is similar to one by Milton H. Erickson (1983).

Erickson states that if you can move the pain to a place in the body where there is no organic cause for it, you can then produce hypnotic anesthesia for the pain at its actual site. You move the patient's subjective experience of the pain to where it does not hurt because you can correct it more easily there. The patient has little resistance to accepting suggestions in the healthy area.

> **In order for a person to experience pain (physical or emotional) to its fullest, the person must give his complete attention to the pain...**
>
> **This places the pain in the role of figure while the other parts of the person that do not hurt, occupy the role of ground.**

In order for a person to experience pain (physical or emotional) to its fullest, the person must give his complete attention to the pain. It seems only natural for anyone to focus attention where it hurts. This places the pain in the role of figure while the other parts of the person that do not hurt occupy the role of ground. The ground (where it doesn't hurt) goes essentially unnoticed. This process can lead to pain magnification or an over-reporting of the experience of pain. In the meantime all the vital resources of the ground go under utilized allowing the pain sufferer to experience maximum pain. The language pattern below invites the person to reverse figure and ground and then associate into the new figure. I will describe a case in which this process proved effective as a method of reducing the experience of pain.

The client presented with physical pain that came about through surgery on his left leg. This procedure relied on a spinal block to deaden the sensation in his leg rather than using a general anesthesia. The spinal block procedure did not turn out well. This caused a problem called Reflex Sympathetic Dystrophy (RSD) a condition that brings considerable pain to the affected areas. For this client, the affected areas included his left foot, parts of his left upper leg and his back.

Please keep in mind if you utilize the hypnotic procedure described below, that the first time you ask the patient to identify where he does *not* hurt, he will usually display the principle of continuation. This often plays out with the client reporting where he *does* hurt because this remains his focus. Repeat your request several times as needed. The hypnotic pattern follows below:

> Raymond, I realize you feel a great deal of pain in your left foot and in your right thigh as well as the middle of your lower back. And I know this hurts a lot. Now, though, I

would like to know where you do not hurt, where do you feel a complete absence of pain? Maybe this includes your ear or your nose or other parts of your body. [*Start by suggesting those places you are most certain he is pain free.*]

Now please take an inventory of sorts, noticing where you feel totally pain free. [*After the first report of an area that is pain free, elicit a state the client associates with being pain free. Then, as the client begins to list the areas where he feels no pain, provide reinforcement with placing the designated state in place of pain free. This client chose the word 'fine' to describe those areas absent of pain.*] Good Raymond, continue noticing and tell me all where you feel fine. [*The closer he gets to the area of actual pain, the more difficult it is for him to find the boundary line. Thus he displays continuation, simplicity and generalization. By focusing on the pain, he displays egocentricity.*]

Now Raymond, what about your right leg, is it completely fine? [*He responds in the affirmative.*] So your whole right leg feels entirely fine, is this right? [*Again, he affirms that he feels fine in his right leg.*] And now Raymond, what parts of your left leg feels fine? [*Ask this question after completing the inventory.*] Now that you notice the parts of you that feel totally fine, what percentage of you would you say feels totally fine, Raymond? [*Raymond responds that 90% of him feels totally fine.*] So Raymond, 90% of you feels 100% fine, 90% of you feels 100% fine, now. How does the 90% of you that feels 100% fine now feel about feeling 100% fine? [*This further dissociates the client from his pain.*]

This process led the client into a state he identified as 'really happy'. I then inquired 'as you remain in this state of really happy, tuned into the part of you that feels 100% fine, what becomes of your pain?' He stated that his pain was nearly gone, just barely noticeable. I received this response from a man who at the first of the session rated his pain as being severe. When he first walked in for the appointment, he had a noticeable limp. When he walked out from the session, he walked with a normal gait.

From that point we went on to strengthen and deepen his ability to shift figure and ground. Also, he learned how to administer mental Novocaine or numbing agents. He reports that at times his pain is completely gone. At other times it is greatly decreased in area and intensity. Also, he has significantly increased his ability to feel emotionally and mentally well.

The Blues: Relieving Depression

In this pattern (as in most others) we follow the steps involved in most successful therapeutic interventions:

1. Associate the client into her problem state—fully experiencing herself.

2. Dissociate the client from her problem state—stepping outside oneself by seeing oneself in the picture.

3. Discover resources—recalling past experiences of resources and/or imagining having them.

4. Associate the client to her resource state—stepping into the resource state and fully experiencing it.

5. Associate resources to the problem state—stepping back into the problem state all the while maintaining the concept of the resource state.

6. Future pace the resource state—imagining moving forward and experiencing the future taking the resources with herself.

Similarity occurs with the use of the word 'blue'. Simplicity and continuation happen when the person experiences the removal of the limiting state and the replacing of it with a resourceful state. This simplifies decision-making because the person can access his resources directly instead of trying to do so while associated into his problem state. We get 'stuck' by associating into our 'stuff' or problem state. We gain resourcefulness and flexibility of behavior by dissociating from our 'stuff'. Continuation automatically happens with each state unless a person consciously chooses not to continue with the same line of thinking.

So you feel like you have the blues, huh? You know I wonder, and you may wonder also, just how the word 'blues' came to be used for feeling down. And just what shade of blue is the blues? Is it dark blue or light blue or does it depend on how low you feel? And why blue and not some other color?

Well maybe you can find some meaning in all this by noticing that blue is also the color of a clear sky. Maybe the blues is sort of a piece of the clear sky that fell out of the clear blue sky and just needs to be replaced, put back up there. Maybe why the blues you have feels bad is because it is out of place. And you can imagine getting this blue and then looking high up into the blue sky, feeling the difference up there.

And notice how this sky seems infinite and really feel the infinite openness and just maybe a piece is missing, the blues you have, so you just put this piece of blue back up where it really belongs, within the infinite. See this to make the clear blue complete and infinite without end. Now how does the clear blue sky feel as you do now as well? Notice the ideas and feelings that now come to you from out of the clear blue sky. And how will you use these now, won't you?

A Carpet of Kindness: Perceiving Your State of Choice

This pattern utilizes the figure-ground, continuation, similarity and dissonance principles. Ericksonian phonological ambiguity occurs with the word 'look', in the second sentence. Similarity also occurs with the use of the phrase 'interior decorating' and 'center piece'. In this pattern, my purpose is to lead the client into noticing, shifting and restoring her choice to both her emotional states as well as perceptual filters.

The rather universal experience of 'room decor' and 'color schemes' serves as the secondary awareness model or metaphor. The person receives an invitation to search through her unconscious mind finding a general memory about 'room décor'. From there the client is led in discovering flexibility of choice through 'interior decorating' as the metaphor that represents her chosen state.

Utilizing the center of the room space also reminds the listener of the usual physical location of most resource states, the center of the person which is usually located in the stomach or chest area. The listener also gets reminded of the infinite range of possibilities through reference to the 'full color spectrum'. The principle of continuation applies to the natural process of continuing to notice like, or similar stimuli in the environment. Continuation and similarity also become the figure, not ground, through suggesting their presence. The principles of continuation and similarity work hand in hand.

> Through the years you certainly noticed different decorating styles in different homes or offices or rooms. Within these spaces you may remember various colors and how several combine to create a particular look…in a certain room containing many colors seeing how one central color, such as in a rug filling the middle of the space, invites you to take notice of similar colors around the room ignoring other, dissimilar colors, even though all the various colors remain. If you replace the certain color rug with a different color rug you can then notice how colors similar to the new rug, previously dormant or in the background, become illuminated.
>
> How interesting, the more you look the more you notice. The more colors present the more opportunity for highlighting the background colors simply by changing the color of the rug. Even colors not in prominence can become more prominent by placing a sort of rallying or organizing point in the center, inviting all similar colors to the forefront. Now you can become your own interior decorator and decide the color for your centerpiece, knowing you can change your centerpiece color any time to highlight different appealing colors for any occasion.
>
> You can place a rug of joy in the center and notice what resonates around it. You can make, as your centerpiece, a rug of eagerness noticing what resonates or a rug of kindness as your centerpiece and notice what resonates. A rug of determination brings all forms of determination to your attention. You may even think of other rugs you want to place for highlighting and creating resonating experiences all around you noticing how you can choose your theme to highlight what you want, now can't you?

Sailing: Identifying and Using Self-Direction

As a NLP Practitioner I (BB) constantly run into adult clients who have the tendency to depend totally on 'external' feedback for everything from decision making to determining how one esteems oneself. Obviously, as children we seek to please our parents and other significant adults. However, as we mature, to continue to depend on 'external' feedback in determining our very identity will lead to co-dependent type behaviors.

> **As we mature, to continue to depend on 'external' feedback in determining our very identity will lead to co-dependent type behaviors.**

Within these words is the message of knowing when and how to switch from external locus of control to an internal, self-directed control. The metaphor used to convey this message is one of a sail-boat and its relationship to the wind and the water. The hypnotic principles employed here include dissonance (pointing out the discrepancy between wanting to move self but not doing so). The pattern also employs egocentrism, as the listener always applies the language pattern to herself. I also employ continuation and simplicity. Similarity takes place with the use of the word 'over-looking'.

Very recently while I was vacationing at the seacoast, I happened to be eating a meal at a restaurant overlooking a harbor. The food was very flavorful and provided to us in a creative way. You know how the chef includes many different colors of food on the plate and it's organized in an artistic way? Well I was eating my meal in the restaurant overlooking the harbor. Not overlooking as in not paying attention to, but overlooking as in paying attention to, with a clear view of the whole scene.

Many boats were docked at the harbor. Some had motors; they were self-propelled. But a lot were sailboats. Several sailboats were in the bay, away from the harbor. The wind blew rather strongly at times and sort of pushed into the sails on the boats making an impression in the sails and propelling the boat.

As my meal went on I noticed that at times the wind decreased leaving the sailboats at a standstill. The sailboats barely moved out in the water. I wondered how the people on the sailboats must feel as the wind died down leaving them sort of adrift. No consistent or persistent direction to their movement they just waited to be moved.

But I also noticed one particular sailboat that did something different from the other sailboats. The people on this sailboat also drifted at first with their boat. But then, after awhile, they took down the sail and went to the back of the boat and started the boat's engine. I thought to myself, 'What a stark contrast in the movement of the boat and the people in it when the boat was propelled by its own engine.'

I then wondered how it must feel being on this boat moving about how you wish, at your own choice, while the others do not. Now you may also wonder what it will feel like when you start up your own engine and propel yourself about, or precisely how you wish toward whatever destination you choose, and how do you know when to start up your engine and where is it you want to go, now? Just listen carefully to the next idea that you harbor.

When it's Over: Addressing Grief

Here I want to address the dynamics of loss and recovery. Grief and joy represent opposite sides of the same coin. When grieving, we rarely, if ever, focus on our future in a joyous way. Instead, we fixate on that which we have lost and the lack of joy. If by chance we should see a future, the grieving person sees nothing but a void created by the loss.

Grief initiates this process as we fixate on the loss in the past. But this process of fixating on the past also deepens grief because by doing so we do not permit ourselves to see new opportunities. Joy comes from invoking the opposite strategy—focusing awareness both on present and future opportunities. As for the loss of the beloved individual, joy preserves the joy of having known the person.

Joy remembers and utilizes the behavioral traits of the departed. Joy wraps around those fond memories of the departed loved one and transforms them into resources for the present and the future. This leads to joy about the continuously available possibilities from that relationship now gone. Essentially this language pattern encourages the person to drop his past and catch the present and future to better honor the loved one.

The principles of similarity and simplicity, as well as continuation, occur throughout this hypnotic pattern. Certainly the foundation for this pattern's effectiveness rests on pointing the person toward a present and future time orientation. Secondary awareness gets invoked when inviting the listener to think about the dynamics of his emotional distress beyond the grief. Asking the listener to consider the consequences of prolonged grief activates a future orientation. This future orientation can then shift to a more resourceful view rather than focusing on the limiting states associated with grief.

It's over when it's over. But how do you know and how do you respond? Not recognizing it's over is like trying to catch a ball already on the ground rather than giving it another go round. Another one is already in the air but stooping to ground level, it just goes over your head. No chance to drop let alone catch.

And just what do you want, mourning or rejoicing, stopping one and starting the other? Know the source of each and that they juxtapose. So how do you detect the over factor? It may be a feeling that begins and you feel you just can't get over it. This one seems easy to catch and hard to drop.

Without specifics, the feeling suggests we look to our past for managing the future. With specifics, we see what we need to do now for the future, which is the opposite. Now catch this one, this means not just catching but looking into the future for the next upcoming opportunity. I hope you catch and hold this one.

Looking into the past means we will look away from our future that holds all we desire. How will you ever... keep from missing the next? You say you were not ready but what were you before you were not ready? Now you're ready.

More clearly than ever knowing exactly what you want because it just went by you and you know the markings... increase your determination for... will... now... anticipate... scanning the horizon... knowing and using.

Small Change: Denominalizing States and Behavior

This pattern came out of a session with a married couple. The wife was engaging in an affair. The couple seemed rather locked into a very rigid pattern of behavior with each other. She could not decide whether or not to end her affair. She knew that if she did not end the affair, she could not focus on saving her marriage, which according to her own report held value to her.

Many rigid beliefs influenced each partner's behavior and the need for flexibility became very important. The pattern itself relies heavily on similarity (*change, metal, mine, give, receive* and *affairs*) and dissonance reduction needs. The use of Phonological Ambiguity creates dissonance. Using such words require the listener to decide what meaning fits the context. Continuation naturally occurs and once shifting takes place, continuation helps keep the shift in place.

The shifting that occurred was specific in some ways and general open-mindedness in others. The more general the shift the more flexibility and broader application it afforded. Specific shifts assist the change process but general shifts carry more flexibility and options.

'I feel a deeper sense of calm throughout my being' incorporates the previous change and carries over into a multitude of other situations. The latter resides at a Meta-level to the former and the Meta change provides a more sweeping reform. The higher the level of change the more influence in the person's life—higher levels modulate lower levels.

This pattern apparently influenced the wife for quite some time after first hearing the pattern. She did, indeed, end the affair and focused on the marriage. She also began loosening her perspective and beliefs. She started 'melting old ways down' in making perceptual changes and continued this process by applying it to other rigid dysfunctional thinking styles.

I saw this client concerning another issue about one year after this session. She initiated reference to this pattern and how it 'just seemed to stick with her' as she considered making other changes. This language pattern lodged within her unconscious mind and she continued effectively applying it in her life.

The words in the hypnotic pattern invite flexibility both in content and process. As we have presented in this work, one of the factors making hypnotic language so effective relates to the cognitive processes involved in interpreting the information within the pattern. The listener must leave behind conventional, concrete thinking, and loosen her cognitive grip on the old patterns. This denominalizes, or melts, frozen processes permitting a 'flow' of consciousness once again.

Interpreting hypnotic language creates a need within the listener to put on her unconscious glasses that will allow the clear reading of new data while at the same time making the old focus fuzzy enough to even disappear. In this sense, figure and ground reverse. The conscious mind shifts from figure to ground and the unconscious mind moves from ground to figure, go figure. The lead in to this pattern calls for reference to 'change' in general.

> As you sit there noticing the chair you sit in and the floor that the chair sits on just allow yourself to let these words sit comfortably in your mind. When you consider making change, you may think about transactions or purchases that produce change, you give and then receive change.
>
> You may also think about the change you now carry in your pocket or purse and what it was before it became your change. Well it was part of the change of the world, it was somebody else's change, it was anybody's change or nobody's change before it became what it was before. It was in a mint being formed and each country can form its own currency or change yet can transform into other's.
>
> Though before it was in a mint it was metal and we shouldn't metal (*meddle*) in anyone else's ... [*Assumes closure of the phrase*

to include in anyone else's … 'affairs, life or business.') And this metal was in a mine or yours … when collected and distributed then melted down to … make change … yet different, yet different in each country and eventually melting down to make new change, aren't you, now?

Recording: Stopping Runaway Strategies

The purpose of these words is to address a former useful process but one that has now extended beyond its effectiveness. The goal involves the listener recognizing the point of diminishing return on a runaway continuation process. Instead of continuing on with old ineffective processes, this pattern encourages the listener in setting boundaries and progressing on toward the goal. The sort of person who may benefit from this pattern is one who gets caught up in the details and loses sight of the bigger picture or purpose.

In this case, due to runaway continuation, details accidentally become figure and overall purpose becomes ground. Suggesting a reversal in this figure-ground relationship makes up the crux of this hypnotic pattern. Using an unwanted outcome and hooking it to the previously believed effective strategy makes the continuation process distasteful, as it becomes counter to overall purpose. A suggested loosening of terms, or lifestyle, occurs in the fourth and fifth sentences. New contents for simplicity and continuation allow future application of the new strategy.

If a person lets her overall purpose drive the decision-making, choices become simpler. Purpose then functions Meta to the details, allowing for Meta-detailing. This process is described in *The Structure of Excellence* (1999):

> The heart and essence of genius (is) the ability to sort for, pay attention to, and recognize details *from a meta-position*. The trained or natural genius has somehow learned to recognize and operate from some meta-pattern or principle that, in turn, allows him or her to see, hear, and sense the richness of details.

> The term *Meta-Details* (and Meta-Detailing) summarizes this gestalt of *small chunking from the perspective of the large chunk.*

A Meta-Detail refers to the crucial and essential details that one can discern and differentiate by using various meta-level distinctions. This means that genius and excellence emerges when we establish a meta-level frame-of-reference that allows us to configure details. (p. 274)

'The heart and essence of genius (is) the ability to sort for, pay attention to, and recognize details from a meta-position.'

Hopefully, by processing the ridiculous nature of the lady in this metaphor as she became consumed with the details, the listener will dissociate from the details and go Meta. From the Meta position, a person can organize the details as to priority and importance. Continuation will just encourage future applications of the simpler process.

The detail-oriented listener may interpret this hypnotic pattern many ways. 'Filling the car with gas' implies preparing for a task but never accomplishing it due to bogging down in details. Also, the listener may just take the words in and realize the need to shift or he may notice how ridiculous it is to continue 'checking the watch'. The listener may get irritated and impatient and simply state how silly it is to keep 'checking the time', saying something like, 'Why doesn't she just pick a time and go!' At this point you reply, 'Yes, that's right' or something to this effect. The listener then 'took the bait' and solved the problem out loud.

I applied this word pattern with a woman who diligently tended to every small detail to the extent that it became difficult for her to accomplish any of her goals. This woman frequently felt frustrated due to her detail-oriented style but also felt compelled to comply with the style believing it so effective.

She would bind herself in the details and then complain about her state of frustration. But beyond the strategy, she really wanted to be an achieving person. Her chosen style prevented this. By amplifying the style and noting the dead end it leads to, she could rise above the style in favor of her stronger desire to achieve desired outcomes. She could attach herself to the desired outcome of her efforts, rather than the step-by-step of how to accomplish, which includes an excess of details.

The client to whom I told this story found the story slightly embarrassing, which verified application to self. But this also provided motivation for change, since the opinion of others mattered to her. She pretty quickly spoke in response to the pattern. She identified ways she could change her detail-oriented style in favor of more streamlined productive methods. She told me what she would now ignore and what she could do instead. She spoke back so quickly that I felt sure her unconscious mind took in the message in the story and replied from awareness. A follow-up visit verified that she decreased the stress in her life by letting go of details and just focusing on achieving her desired outcomes.

> This is a story about a person who likes things well organized. She keeps track of every little detail so she can know exactly what's going on. She even extends this process to how she gets gasoline in her car. It may seem strange but she actually has a detailed process for how and what to do in filling her car with gas, well the gas tank actually, not the whole car.

> Sometimes things get taken literally and that can be confusing. Looser terms, you know, can be easier and more effective. So each time she fills the car with gas she records the mileage, the number of gallons she got and then calculates the miles per gallon. She recently decided to also record the time of day or night she gets the gasoline, this just to be more precise in her records. You can't know too much, you know?

> But here comes the problem. The first time she decided to use her new method of including the time of day she got the gasoline the trouble began. She sits in her car after filling the tank and begins recording. When she gets to the part of recording time she feels the confusion setting in like a permanent passenger. At first she wrote down the time but then looked at her watch a second time just to be sure she recorded the right time and found her watch showed a different time. It was a few seconds beyond the time she recorded.

> In the name of precision, she erased and rewrote the new time. Now double checking her watch she found it showed another new time. Well, erasing again with bits of rubber flying along with old led her back to rewrite the now more

accurate time. But double-checking the time led her to realize she was inaccurate once again.

The precise person who is so focused on everything being perfectly organized never did anything else ever again because time always continues. In the name of time she got lost in it and what will happen when she leaves time out?

The Bridge That Is: Remembering Purpose to Motivate Constructive Action

This hypnotic language pattern takes the form of an extended metaphor. This intense metaphor emphasizes the benefit of goal-oriented perception and behavior as well as the consequences for abandoning purpose. I suggest that you do not use this story with anxiety prone clients or with those who lack motivation.

The target audience of this pattern includes those with high motivation who tend to get caught up in details and get bogged down losing sight of their original purpose. These people just need to get on top (meta-level) of their mental processes and move on rather than remaining stalled in the quicksand of details. Utilizing an away-from or avoidance strategy, this pattern seeks to un-stick the stuck. It intends to render the 'why question' mute, permitting refocusing on the desired outcome which will result in the client progressing towards her goal.

Asking 'why' more often than not seeks justification for present behavior rather than discovering the higher purpose of behavior. This is explained in *The User's Manual for the Brain* (1999):

> That point which is how the question 'Why?' often involves Cause-Effect ill-formedness. Dennis and Jennifer Chong, in their thought provoking book, *Don't Ask Why: A Book about the Structure of Blame, Mad Communication and Miscommunication*, point out that often when we ask the question 'Why?' we are in fact looking for reasons and explanations. They conclude that, 'Once you have the *reason* or *explanation*, you have the *cause*. You know what *made* you do it. The questions 'Why?' therefore seeks the elucidation of the relationship between two classes of variables or things: the class of variables that are the cause and the class of variables that are the effects'

172

(page 81). Thus, asking 'Why?' rather than looking for solutions to the problem will often deepen the problem by eliciting reasons and justification. (pp. 144–45)

> **'Asking "Why?" rather than looking for solutions to the problem will often deepen the problem by eliciting reasons and justification.'**

In order to 'un-stick' the 'stuck' we need to direct their attention away from the 'why' of 'details' and towards the higher purpose. This pattern seeks to do that.

Once, once, just once, there…was a man who wanted to go from point A to point R. He wanted point R to be what is. He found himself on one side of a piece of land. This is point A. On the other side is a piece of land that is point R. Point A and point R are separated by a deep, deep, *deeeep…chasm*. And the distance between the two sides extends too far to leap across. This man wants very much to get across the chasm to point R. He longs for this moment. So he begins walking, rapidly at first and then even faster, to find a way across the chasm, the deep, deep, *deeep…chasm*. His walking is fueled by his desire, need, wanting and longing to be on the other side.

He walks at terrific speeds all along the banks of this piece of land. Looking, looking for a place where the chasm may not be as deep or as wide. Days pass and he grows hungry, tired and thirsty since he's barely had any food or drink for days. Yet his hunger to get across the chasm far exceeds the hunger he feels in his stomach. A far greater emptiness exists within. His travels take him from the rather sparse flatlands to the more plush woods. He remains determined to find a way across.

While walking early one morning, after barely any rest, he sees a vague outline of a structure off in the distance. He cannot fully make out the image. The closer he gets the more he sees and yet the more he can't believe what he thinks he sees. This may be the answer to his pleading and praying. It's a bridge.

This long arching wooden bridge extends fully across the chasm touching down on the other side. This is truly amazing. The wooden bridge appears old but looks solid. It may well be safe to cross, leading him to his long awaited fulfillment. Wow! This is almost too good to be true. With a surge of energy about the possibilities, he approaches and takes a closer look at the bridge.

The bridge consists of thick wooden planks and sturdy looking supports piercing into the ground. How is this bridge … what holds this bridge together? Nails? … and just how … and who? Do more exist? This is quite an amazing sight for the very tired walker. A rush of curiosity-driven questions arise. Well it is time to actually step onto the bridge to find out if it will hold up his wishes.

His first sort of tentative step finds a solid feeling support with no shaking underneath. Now both feet bring his full weight to bear on the structure. Not the first creak or bend. Now he could more closely examine the planks running across the structure that provides the walking surface. He tries to identify the type of tree the planks come from. He looks closely but gets no clear answer for this question.

He continues walking carefully and alertly. Gosh, even sturdy handrails along this bridge. Who would think of such things? Wow! And look at the view that comes into focus from even the first few feet of the hundred or so to the other side. He looks down to the very bottom of the chasm. How small things look down there.

He next looks down the length of the chasm finding a winding stream flowing through it. He wonders if fish swim in the stream and what kinds of plants grow in the basin. He continues sort of gazing and meandering on the bridge gradually moving up the incline toward the crest.

All the while he notices the variations in the wood grain and the views of the distance the bridge affords him, looking near, looking far. He observes how each piece of wood is cut with smooth, straight, precise lines. Each fits together with the next forming a line to walk across. He observes the weathering that took place on the wood, different at different places depending on the degree of exposure to the elements. Very consistent it appears.

His fascination continues as he observes how all these pieces and parts present themselves combining into such an amazing structure, and just who and how. He just stares at the bridge with great wonder, so many questions and so much intrigue.

He feels so spent but now renewed by what he discovered. He slowly steps one foot after another foot along the wooden surface. He continues taking in so many details with great fascination. The views from above, parallel to the bridge, and now these strange markings he sees etched into the wood.

All along the handrails and even on the walking surface, some sort of carving marked into the wood, each the same familiar design. This sure draws him in for a closer look. Down on his hands and knees to get a close look he not only sees the design but with each, an inscription. Looking up and out along the surface, these markings dot the wood as far as he can see.

Once looking at just one of the designs he determines the marking is a cross, not across but a cross, consisting of two lines intersecting to form the sign of a cross. Underneath this one is someone's name and a date in the distant past. The next cross that's carved into the wood also has a name and date underneath it.

Each one he inspects carries a name and date underneath it. These dates range from hundreds of years old to the fairly recent past. Widening his view, literally hundreds of crosses, each with names and dates, litter the wooden surface. Now beginning to shake with emotion at the sheer volume, he freezes in his hands and knees position. What does this all mean?

By now the light of early day gives way to the early evening indirect light. He spent nearly all day examining and inspecting the bridge, the views afforded and now the obsession with the crosses and their significance. Were these some sort of memorial to people who died here on this bridge? And why so many people perishing on this bridge over so many hundreds of years?

After sunset now with dusk settling in he suddenly hears some rustling coming from the edge of the woods just behind him. He turns to look and sees a particular animal emerging from the woods. This animal is known as a gostalk and only hunts in the dark because of its night vision. Fast and ferocious, this animal searches for meat and fears nothing. It is an animal on a mission.

Well, investigating the bridge comes to an immediate halt. Now he must slip quickly and silently across the bridge before the gostalk notices him and attacks. He quietly moves over the crest of the arched bridge and gets his first glimpse of the other half. Terror fills him like water from a broken dam. There at the point where the bridge touches down on the other side of the chasm stands a gostalk. Now he knows.

Questioning: Preventing Anger

This pattern unexpectedly resulted in the context of an active session. It came about as a sort of natural phenomenon—it just came out of my unconscious mind. The client, Darrin, displayed the response being described in the language pattern. No doubt my unconscious mind knew what was going on but my conscious mind remained in the dark.

Darrin presented with a problem of bringing his hot temper under control. He often flew into a rage at the least provoking and expressed his anger at his new wife—not good. While he displayed the rage response during the dating and engagement period, his rage response increased shortly after the marriage.

The process of becoming angry or the more amplified version called 'rage', often involves jumping to conclusions. I believe anger bases itself on fear of losing worth or esteem. The person generates such a degree of fear over the imagined loss that he must then defend himself with anger. But the key step in the process requires the angry person to jump to conclusions. This leap puts the person in the place of feeling his self-worth or self-esteem is in danger of being lost.

Darrin also easily jumped to conclusions, fearing loss of worth in the eyes of his new spouse. The pattern below addresses his tendency to jump to conclusions and then identifies an alternative

—his asking questions to collect information. I asked the client to describe a specific incident of his rage so I could then apply the hypnotic pattern. I also made sure he identified the first signal he received from his wife that served as the trigger for him to feel angry. He reported this occurs in his gut. This initial signal will later come to serve as the cue to switch tracks to a different response rather than going down the dead-end anger track.

He described a trigger from a recent series of experiences with his wife in which he took some limited information from his wife and then plugged in his many assumptions. This immediately resulted in a state of intense anger. During these anger episodes he seemed inconsolable and immune to reasoning. The angry emotions were outframing (moving outside) his reasoning abilities. Usually he needed two or three days to reset to some sort of emotional balance. Once he described the incident I then spoke the short pattern below.

The pattern involves changing the meaning of his anger and reframing it into a useful state that would lead to a solution. Some simplicity principle gets used along with the ever-present continuation. In this case, simplicity refers to removing the complicated layers that follow the jumped-to conclusion, fear, rage and the emotional 'clean up' after the fight. Replacing the complex steps with just simple information gathering questions allows a more simplified approach to an issue. This pattern relies almost exclusively on the dissonance reduction drive, the drive to match beliefs with behavior. But the effectiveness also relies on the client's values.

This client placed significant value on the relationship becoming more pleasant and constructive. Because of this, the dissonance reducing would result in emphasizing the welfare of the relationship. By emphasizing the importance of the relationship, the events that triggered his anger would lose its power. Because of his natural emphasis on preserving the relationship, I made sure to praise this and amplify his priorities. This made it an easier choice (simplification) of releasing his anger in exchange for behaviors that resulted in more marital harmony.

So Darrin, when you start to feel this anger that you report starts in your gut, maybe what you find there is not anger but rather confusion. And if this is really confusion, then won't asking questions in the process of assembling conclusions bring the answers you seek and will it work best if you start asking these questions at the very first awareness of this confusion so you can get the information right away allowing relief as soon as possible?

Immediately after I spoke these words, Darrin remained silent for just a second or two and then spoke. He asked, 'So what you mean is that I just listen to others and then ...' At this point I cut him off and said, 'Exactly!!' verifying emphatically that he was demonstrating the idea perfectly as he sat there asking me this question. He looked puzzled for just a couple of seconds and then his eyes darted back and forth as he processed. He then smiled and proudly proclaimed that he now got it. He went right back into trance and re-calculated and then proclaimed how he understood now. He just continued sitting there in sort of stunned amazement looping back through the thought sequence several more times quietly saying how he now understood it.

Follow-up several weeks later with both the husband and wife verified that the client no longer displayed temper outbursts. Instead he engaged in a series of questions that permitted an effective discussion of concerns. He no longer felt the urge to go into a rage and found his new style helped create the desired relations between his wife and himself.

Taste Tester —*Paralysis of Analysis*

This story addresses the person who suffers from 'paralysis of analysis'. This type of person has much difficulty moving forward due to the need for analyzing in an attempt to gather enough information so it is 'safe' to move forward.

> **As you know, a person can either experience or analyze an experience but cannot do them simultaneously.**

As you know, a person can either experience or analyze an experience but cannot do them simultaneously. The 'experiencing position' essentially associates the person into state. You may think of this in time orientation as living immersed in the moment—a full participator in the event in the current time. In NLP we refer to this person as living 'in time', i.e. in the moment. The 'analytical position' dissociates the person placing them in the 'through time' perspective. Think of the 'through time' perspective as a detached position of an observer noticing events from a slight distance.

As we have discussed, for change in states, beliefs or behavior to happen, the person must first step into (associate) the problem state: second, the person must step outside (dissociate) the problem state; third, the person will discover and step into (associate) the resource state; and, fourth, the person will hold the resource state and bring it to bear onto the problem state (associate resources to the problem). Remaining on the sidelines in the analytical perspective prevents change since the person never associates into or commits to a resource state or belief.

> **Remaining on the sidelines in the analytical perspective prevents change since the person never associates into or commits to a resource state or belief.**

The following hypnotic language pattern or short tale addresses the limiting side effects of the analytical perspective and encourages an experiential position. The story also addresses the suspicious or fearful state that gives rise to the safer feeling analytical perspective. It does so by pointing the person to the dangers of her away–from strategy that avoids associating into experiential-action states. The only experience going on for the analytical person is analysis. This person tends to remove herself from interacting with life and only interacts with information. She resists converting information into goal-oriented action. I (BB) have observed that many over-analytical type people find state association most uncomfortable. So, they live dissociated, where it 'feels' safe.

This story takes place back in the days of knights. In these days many dangers exist for those in power positions. Many other people seem to want to overthrow those who rule. For this reason the ruling body often employs what is known as taste testers. These people have the job of tasting all foods prior to the ruler and other important persons eating.

This is done because often the easiest way to kill off someone in power is through poisoning the food of the rulers. If a tester does not sample the food first then analyze it for taste and, of course, stay alive, the ruler and important others could be in danger by eating the food before the taste tester. So the job of the taste tester is simply to eat some food and consider its worth and then let a little time pass to prove that the food is not poisoned.

It may seem simple enough but one taste tester somehow got the necessary order reversed. Rather than tasting and then analyzing, this taster tried to analyze before eating, being such an analytical person you know. Well everyone, including the ruler, kept waiting for results but there is nothing to analyze without first tasting.

The head of state pleads with and then tries to force the taste taster to find out if the food is edible. And by now several meals have come and gone with potentially hunger-satisfying food spoiling, going to waste. Everyone continues getting hungrier and hungrier. Well this process continues, of analyzing before tasting thus having nothing to analyze, and the whole royal family starves to death including the taste tester! What a waste, you know?

The Last Thing You Would Think: Accessing Resources and Keeping Them

The words in this language pattern rely on the principle of continuation from Gestalt psychology. The concept and process of figure-ground also play a role in this hypnotic pattern. The idea here is to access the continuation and figure-ground principles and then to apply them to states that promote resourceful responses.

> **Reversing the figure-ground arrangement allows previously ignored information-resources to come into awareness, which will create new possibilities.**

Reversing the figure-ground arrangement allows previously ignored information-resources to come into awareness, which will create new possibilities. The stimuli associated with sustaining a resource state receive highlighting. This will cause the resource state stimuli to come into consciousness or to become the figure.

By this, I mean the person will notice choices that remain consistent with the resource-state and ignore choices that create dissonance within the state. Also, the natural tendency for people to continue noticing themes that they have already noticed encourages sustaining the resource state. The listener will continue on the lookout for opportunities.

Human nature, certain ways about humans seem undeniable. Many researchers and scientists study and document these most natural of styles we humans possess. This leads to one in particular. The tendency to find repeating repeating patterns based on the content of your last experience. Have you ever read a book or seen a show and then went on about your business? And then did you notice how you tended to find the same topics or themes as the recently noticed material in the next several situations. And this may involve any of the five senses?

It is almost as though what you most recently encounter provides a lens through which to experience the world for a time. You just notice similar themes, more of the same. Now the preceding experience tinting your perceptions must stand out enough to make an impact on you.

You must believe the material useful or significant to you in order to make a lasting impression. This plays out when you buy a car that's new to you. Almost immediately after, you notice all the similar cars. It is as though these cars are illuminated or standout in some way, while the rest of the cars fade into the background.

As humans, we apparently attempt continuing a pattern if it seems significant to us. And of course now you know this and will find that you begin doing this process but find it more conscious because these very words become one of the examples it concerns. We could go even deeper, you know.

And now you may even begin wondering what this article will end up on, making this the last thing you think thus sending you on a can't miss mission noticing other examples of the last thing you think. Maybe it will end on a high note referring to some most desirable state or trait. Maybe it will finish what it started leading to satisfaction.

And it could stop at the point where you simply become aware that you find what you are aware of so chose what you want to be aware of and you will find this is so. [*The therapist can follow this last sentence up with asking the listener what she wants to become aware of and find, now.*]

Becoming Is: Shifting From One State into Another

In this pattern I utilize a sort of double mirror process. At the same time I explain the dynamics of 'becoming' a particular state, I apply a state that seems to increase receptivity and enthusiasm. So, in effect, the listener receives an invitation to become enthusiastic and then, this same state is used.

The hypnotherapist will want to apply the pattern to the individual's specific situation. The words also point out that since most states of mind pre-exist, a person can choose his states rather than concerning himself with creating them. The reference to 'planet' (last paragraph) suggests to the listener to 'plan it' (similarity).

> **The logic in this pattern involves the principle that naming a state, results in natural associating into, or, at least being aware of it from a dissociated position.**

The last part uses what I believe represents another form of hypnotic language—logic. The logic in this pattern involves the principle that naming a state results in natural associating into it, or at least being aware of it from a dissociated position. The pattern leads the listener down the path and then reaches the inevitable double bind conclusion.

Just by answering the question, yes or no, the listener will verify the preceding logic train because the listener must process the question to answer it. While confusing to the conscious mind, processing the question and contemplating answers gets the listener in contact with choice—the very principle presented within the language pattern.

This process is like asking someone if he is thinking about the color blue right now. To answer this question, the listener must think about the color blue and then, either keep it on his mind, or shift to another subject. But for at least a brief moment, he accessed the color you wanted him to consider. So it is with this pattern, the listener at least has to consider and try on the ideas you present. Now he can continue operating from enthusiastic choice, that is, if he chooses to do so.

> The words making up language possess some intriguing qualities. While words you hear remain invisible they carry certain properties. Even though they exist, they are also inanimate, just products of our imagination in a sense. Yet these words also contain a kind of ability to evoke feelings in the speaker and listener.

> Feelings, in this case, refer to both emotions and physical sensations. In particular, notice how certain words generate a physical response when hearing them. For example, the word enthusiasm stirs an energy source within. You may need to draw upon past memories of enthusiasm to remember if some time passed since last feeling enthusiasm. If it has been a while since you last felt enthusiasm you may find yourself experiencing enthusiasm enthusiasm. Now you have it don't you?

> Now think about the word becoming, an especially interesting word that seems forever evolving. It acts almost like a train engine propelling whatever rests in front of it toward its destination. When you are becoming you are yet to get there, and when you get there you are no longer becoming, you are there. Yet the result may be becoming to you, if you get what I say.

What are you becoming, either slowly or quickly what will you be when you get there, no longer becoming but being, now? Choose your desire, deeply feeling then becoming brings to the surface the very you want to be using now, aren't you? And when you are becoming realize you move toward what already exists.

You would see no destination if it did not already present itself in response to your request. So you become what you want, right? While you adjust your form or style you do not create a truly new style overall but move to a style already existing like a.... planet, discovered only after its presence in the present. So you can decide what you want to discover and become this now because to decide is to name and to name is to know and to know is to become, isn't this so now? And just by answering the question you have verified this.

Critical Mistake: Limiting and Eliminating Self-Criticism

The principles addressed here include figure-ground, continuation, similar states of emotion and perceptual filters in general. The metaphor of containing an oil spill compares to a strategy for reacting to personal mistakes. Many references occur to the area not contaminated and utilizing the double meaning of sea/see (similarity, phonological ambiguity) occurs several times to invoke visual representation making a fuller and more effective experience.

The figure becomes all uncontaminated parts of self—the clean that comprises the vast majority of the self. The spill becomes ground, making it less influential. The containing of the spill isolates the unpleasant emotional state and limits its influence on other parts of self. By referring to the clean and clear parts of the water, i.e. the self, the individual receives an invitation to associate into resourceful positions at broader and deeper levels. In general, the words take the listener through the process of associating into the problem-state, dissociating from it and then associating into resourceful states.

I applied this hypnotic pattern in a case with a man who frequently felt depressed after judging he made some sort of error. This man, in his early 40s, was highly self-critical. Many factors from his past contributed to creating his style. But by this time in his life, his current thoughts represented the only factor that sustained the self-critical pattern. He generalized from one error to then judge himself harshly in all facets of his life.

> **He exemplified the truth that beliefs function as self-organizing systems attracting from the environment those situations, that sustain their existence.**

He constantly remained on the lookout for any other possible mistakes. He thus exemplified the truth that beliefs function as self-organizing systems attracting from the environment those situations that sustain their existence. He took all mistakes personally, which led to his believing himself as being incompetent. As a point of fact, this man owned a very successful home construction business and employed many people including the vast majority of his extended family.

When he came in for counseling he presented as quite depressed. It became clear the problem stemmed from contaminated thinking that led him to feel depressed and worthless. After talking with him and eliciting how he depressed himself, a fairly distinct thought pattern and process emerged. This hypnotic language pattern offered a coping mechanism as well as a replacement thought process in place of the erroneous thinking styles he presently engaged in.

Once hearing the content and process, he immediately found the concept appealing and noted how it would help him limit his runaway critical thinking. The focus shifted from his supposed behavioral error to the thought response within him that led to this erroneous thinking. His thinking styles that depressed him repre-sented the only true mistake, a critical mistake. This now could be cordoned off and limited.

After this session of hearing and installing the new response style, he returned to the next session reporting significant improvement. He now knew he could control his thoughts by treating them from a sort of detached or dissociated position. This limited his self-critical thinking and he ultimately removed the contaminated ones replacing them with cleaner, clearer thoughts. Several weeks later this man reported he continued feeling well and contained any 'spills' quickly and easily. He also reported that he had resumed enjoying some of his hobbies that he had given up because he was trying to prove his competence even in his hobbies.

> What happens when you treat any mistake, and every mistake, like an oil spill at sea? First see the sea and the spill area. Then place the barriers around the oil containing the spill. Now remember and notice how the ocean outside the containers remains clear and clean.

> Also remember that oil is lighter than water so it floats, resting only on the surface. The water underneath the oil also remains clear and clean. Now the only task remaining is removing, skimming the oil from the sea... see it disappear slowly or quickly noticing the feeling as the oil leaves more and more sea to see and feel... the clear and clean return. Now, how will you enjoy the sea sight as you set your sights on your future?

Chapter Seven

Language Patterns Addressing Spiritual Matters

In this chapter we utilize hypnotic language patterns in addressing spiritual issues. This collection aims to access what, we believe, holds the most humbling and comforting power an individual may access—her spirituality. We realize that not everyone holds or believes in any form of spirituality. However, at the same time, a large number do. And, it is for these that we include this short chapter. For the reader who does not hold any specific religious beliefs, we invite you to access your higher values whatever they may be as you process these patterns.

Some of the power available from the spiritual realm stems from the awareness of being connected to the larger whole, both within the individual as a person and, more powerfully, to the whole of the universe. But, does any difference exist between the two? To know one is to know the other. These hypnotic language patterns remind you that, as humans, we simply represent a tangible form of the intangible spiritual world, both an honor and an opportunity.

> **These hypnotic language patterns remind you that, as humans, we simply represent a tangible form of the intangible spiritual world, both an honor and an opportunity.**

As humans we encounter so many distractions that we tend to forget our origins and purpose. These language patterns serve to remind, refresh, reassure and support the original purpose with renewed vigor. The ultimate purpose of these words is the total removal of the sense of 'pressure' and then to reconnect the individual to her concept of spirituality where 'safety' dwells. This type of thinking permits a much more effective conceptual lifestyle. These hypnotic language patterns almost exclusively rely on simply accessing secondary awareness or the unconscious mind through expanding awareness. For, it is in our unconscious mind where one can access those high level spiritual states that promote a sense of 'safety' and 'congruency' with one's world.

> **These hypnotic language patterns almost exclusively rely on simply accessing secondary awareness or the unconscious mind through expanding awareness.**

Ambassador: Humans Representing the Spirit of Purpose

The words in this pattern represent several concepts. The concepts include the ideas of a 'purposeful existence' and 'clarity' of this purpose. While we may believe we know our purpose, enacting this can become confusing at times. Encouraging a purposeful existence and clarity of purpose occurs in the reference to utilizing gifts or internal resources that each of us possess. Emphasis is placed on utilizing the gifts rather than getting caught up in tracking down the source of the gifts.

The last two lines in the pattern about whom to provide with help also play a role of clarifying life's purpose. The third principle addressed is the person existing as an extension of many supportive beings under the protective umbrella of a Supreme Being. These words and concepts also aim to create a calm, yet certain state of determination for carrying out the designed purpose. Inviting secondary awareness occurs throughout this language collection.

> You represent many people, seen and unseen. Some you know and some you have yet to know. Not unlike the dwelling you now occupy, many previous occupants spent time there. They each leave behind traces of themselves and their lives that influence. You are here now but where were you before and where will you go later, yet right on time? There is only one common denominator.
>
> Some say your 'personality' stems from your DNA while others say your 'personality' results from a chemical reaction process, environment interacting with you and vice-versa.

Maybe what we refer to as 'personality' is just what we show to others the most. But what we show differs within and between only representing a small fraction of the whole.

How many different four-number combinations can be made with 100 numbers? Well there is a formula for figuring such and the total is astounding, I know this much. Now, how many 2, 3, 4 or more number combinations can you make with several thousand numbers, and now with the infinite that is? Such is your personality.

When you express any trait, it must, by necessity, take an observable form. It could not be gathered or displayed otherwise. But this status is temporary, only for the time in use. Don't be fooled by the one or two forms on display because the immense intangible lot remains in waiting, yet weightless. All traits waiting in the wings naturally take a non-form yet they inform, remaining adaptable. Don't let out of sight become out of mind.

So what is your 'personality'? Well, in a sense you are an ambassador representing so much and so many. You choose the best, suiting the cause, supported by many. What you choose to represent is your 'personality'. Therefore, your 'personality' is simply an outward expression of your purpose.

Input comes from an inner circle yet this just represents the whole collection of circles. You get the tangible while the rest is intangible. If you make it your purpose to identify where you got what you have you will not be able to have what you got. You are an ambassador, representing a significant collective, quite a privilege. Always dispatched by the high command, you arrive with a support staff though most work behind the scenes. Do not fear those whom you have come to help, help those who have come to fear. The task then remains clear.

Appreciation: Appreciating the Ultimate Resource

The first part of this pattern simply asks the listener to go into trance. The initial trance is general and then the client is invited into a more specific trance of appreciation. This invitation happens by going into detail about a universal human phenomenon that noticing details begets more noticing of details. Listening to the explanation of this process in the hypnotic pattern allows the development of a trance. Now that the unconscious mind becomes available to the speaker and listener, directing this to useful awareness makes up the second step.

The words in this pattern suggest that to achieve desired outcomes, a person most needs to access and use her unconscious mind. Also identified are the dangers of mistaking self rather than spirituality (referred to as 'not self' in the pattern) as the source of accomplishments and the undesirable outcome associated with this self-centered process. The two parts, accessing and then using the unconscious mind provide a sort of team energizing the person in the desired direction.

> Now you know that when you notice something and pay full attention to it, closing out all other awareness, you can only then fully appreciate the full depth of something. And, in fact, the more you notice after closing out all other awareness, the more you notice about the one thing you pay full attention to, don't you? Now noticing even more please allow yourself to notice that when you fully notice your sources of knowing you find that they reside in a form called *not self*. Self only exists as a conduit so you can do it.

> Don't be fooled into believing that your self accomplished any act on its own other than paying attention to the *not self*. This *not self* contains not one thing, it *contains everything*. When you believe your self is the source you then pay attention to your self. Then what do you not pay attention to—the *not self*. This resembles living off the limitations of your short-term memory or surviving from just a canteen filled with water rather than the infinite source of the water, freely dipping and filling.

> Focusing on self prevents new awareness and limits the extent of knowledge and skills, sealing them off from the life-giving sources, permanently limiting and dooming to eventual extinction. Recognize and remember how you developed awareness in the past, tuning in to the infinite spring and continuing this process allows continuing awareness of what you now know is new. And you want to k-n-o-w more now, don't you? Just appreciate the connection

and experience the free flow noticing the difference between receiver and sender.

One For the Ages: *Recognizing and Experiencing Eternal Resources*

The words in this pattern attempt to provide a deeper or higher sense of awareness of concepts and principles that exist on a permanent basis in this universe. People who focus externally too much set themselves up for insecurity. They also set themselves up for inevitable loss and grief. Internally focused people are likely to recover from loss more easily as they access their internal resources rather than bemoaning those lost resources through another departed person, being or thing.

> **People who focus too much externally set themselves up for insecurity.**

The pattern below aims to remind and restore the person to an internal focus on those concepts that remain eternally present, never changing over time—love, peace, harmony, happiness and security represent some of the elements universally available on a permanent basis. This collection represents the elements that provide comfort and allow a person to choose effectively in life.

Existing as a tangible being, it becomes all too easy to forget our intangible inner self and seek tangible means in the pursuit of feeling good. But these tangible means are fleeting, just as we are. Remembering, accessing and utilizing the positive intangible resources permit a person to truly find and experience the desired outcome first. Once choosing the outcome, the individual can more healthily choose the proper actions or behaviors for himself. One then naturally chooses actions in keeping with the sense of peace, love and/or safety.

Yes, you are right, everything does age and grow older. Nothing seems to last forever, nothing tangible that is. All things you can see, touch, smell, taste or... hear... your senses know that all they perceive is fleeting and eventually disappears. From the moment something of a tangible nature comes into existence it begins deteriorating. Even the book containing the concepts and ideas in tangible form decays. Its only purpose is to convey or transfer certain ideas to others.

But the really amazing fact is that some things never age no matter how old they are. Does the concept of *love* grow old? Does the concept of *peace* age? How about *total security*, does this idea or place of the idea ever age? *Total security is totally secure.* All things in your imagination or that you experience never age. When you think about peace, love and total security, do you realize these ideas and this awareness existed forever?

We as humans, are born, age and then we die. But there are intangible concepts that never age. I wonder who you think gave birth to these ageless wonders that remain forever available for us. And maybe you are like the book, just here for others to receive certain ideas and concepts. I wonder what you want and will convey to others. Of course your contents sort of determine what you convey.

So consider these ageless concepts that provide such continuous availability and what do you feel when you know that this is so you can know that these ideas and experiences never age making for continuous security of peace, love and total safety. Not created by humans thus can't be affected by humans, just experienced and conveyed. All that exists in tangible form exists temporarily.

Consider a foundation made from the intangible concepts that never age and notice the certainty. How will this allow you to rely on these sound ideas and use them from moment to moment, second to second, first? What does this awareness convey to you to convey in your life, now?

Know Your Woods: *Taking Actions Based on Faith and Trust*

This pattern utilizes a concept inherit in most of the world's religions—the concepts of 'trust' and 'faith.' Trust and faith seem to function opposite to that of doubt. Certainly, in the Judeo/Christian belief structures, this is true. Faith and trust give a person access to unlimited resources within.

The words utilize similarity (similarity automatically invokes confusion, or dissonance, and then the next point of reference presented becomes that to which the listener latches on to). The pattern also utilizes continuation several times by inviting the listener to elevate her levels of trust and faith.

The following pattern relies on the principle of similarities for part of its effect. But the similarity in this case stems from the American pronunciation of the words 'dew' and 'do'. Therefore, the pattern may only be useful with those clients who use an American pronunciation.

> It seems what makes the difference at the deepest levels comes down to faith. But what is faith built on because you must have something going between the tangible world and the place of faith, intangible. Faith seems built on a bridge made of trust wood. And in the early light you can see the dew on it and looking closer allows you to feel the *dew*. If you get there even earlier you can see the *dew* making *dew*, *dewing*, what it knows best.

> Always at the right time, the dew point. If dew comes down followed by more dewing then you get 2 *dew*. And notice how all parts receive the dew equally. It's probably best when all parts get 2 *dews*. It's even more. And now that you are there, hear… the *dew*… you can even feel the faith filling you to become faithful.

> Now knowing this feeling you can notice how it provides fuel to move you toward what you want, and you know what you want, now, don't you…. keep your eyes and ears on the goal only noticing how to adjust allowing you to continue moving toward your goal… that you set your sights on.

Three Part Harmony: Working in Harmony with the Spirit

The words within this collection relate to the three necessary elements present in any event. First there must exist an object or stimulus. This object or stimulus then receives stimulation from a second object, or stimulus. The stimulation may come in the form of perceiving or of a more active interacting. Representing the third part present in any event is the interaction by-product. This takes the form of the thought, behavior or state of mind-emotion. A person interacts with his environment and the result is a thought. This thought leads to emotions and behavior.

An entity existing alone in a vacuum exists in a steady state. Once a second stimulus interacts with the first, a reaction occurs. The language pattern below describes this three-part process and then relates it to the spiritual domain. If the three parts actor, stimulus and action exist in harmony, producing constructive purposeful actions, then a three-part harmony occurs. On the highest plane, the listener may view the three parts as Supreme Being, self and the actions inspired by making oneself a conduit to the Supreme Being. This results in the ultimate three-part harmony.

> You know there are many references to three in various circles. We eat three meals a day. While this makes a triangle we refer to the meals as squares so it is sort of a square within a triangle if you can picture this. We have three names, first, middle and last. Vocalists perform in three-part harmony. And on a deeper level, you can find three parts to the change process.

> There is the current style and then the place you go to in order to get away from the now old way, a transition you know, and then you come up to the third part, that is the new way, the change, you know. It is sort of three realities always available at any one time, if you can imagine this.

> In order to take out the trash you have to go from a position before holding the trash to picking it up and then letting it go in the right place at the right time. The third part of the three is the most crucial, letting go of the trash, washing your hands, then picking up whatever you desire now.

> You can also be aware of the three parts playing a role in any thought you experience. The external event or general stimulus, the awareness of it then the meaning attributed. The threes combine to make-up the process resulting in any belief. Just like the flower bulb planted underground. It knows where it is at all times and considers the place and time then consults its purpose, to bloom. The next thing you know the bulb believes it's time to emerge from the buried depths, up through the layers until going above the ground level to fully bloom.

Actions spring from beliefs. All beliefs take into account the external situation, your own purpose and then actions occur accordingly, a three-part process. And if the belief ignores the purpose a felt loss of purpose through impulse occurs but not on purpose. And if the belief ignores the external then another loss occurs, flexibility becomes rigidity, losing ultimate purpose.

The third outcome is a harmonious one considering purpose along with external conditions for an inclusive belief. In addition to purpose and beliefs is the part conducting the whole process creating three-part harmony. This conductor knows the score. You may believe other elements bring about our beliefs. This may be so yet many and, in fact, all things may be so. We just choose the beliefs we believe best serve our purpose, don't we? Either way you answer it's true, don't you believe?

The preceding principle reminds me of a person I once knew from the past who stated he could not be himself. This is like saying you can make music without an instrument. You know you can only produce music if you have an instrument and a violin cannot sound like a trumpet. No music is heard without an instrument, be it percussion, wind or string.

Here, you find another three-part collection comprising the whole. And yet each of these in its simplest form is really just a form of percussion, one element coming in contact with another. This may be wind moving across a gap, a finger or bow contacting string or object meeting object.

So the three are really one. One contacting one, producing music or even any sound you hear the three are of one but all require three. No single element can sound without another to interact with and some result is only natural. It cannot not make a sound reaction. What sound do you desire to make and with what instruments are you an instrument of making three-part harmony here? You see?

Universe: Entering Any 'State' You Choose

This language in the pattern seeks to invoke a tone of spiritual awareness within the listener. The purpose of the pattern is to assist the listener by relieving his feelings of aloneness. The only way to occupy a sense of aloneness essentially involves a disregard of secondary awareness. The words below relate to accessing the listener's secondary awareness and then extend this beyond to the sense of oneness between all, not just within.

The only way to occupy a sense of aloneness essentially involves a disregard of secondary awareness.

The connecting satisfies the closure-wholeness need and the inclusion need. Because if the inclusion need is not met, then the person is not whole, but not knot hole, go figure. From here the process moves to considering free access to and associating into any state of his choice—the grand design of all resources existing within for our use.

The perspective taken and expressed in the pattern is that states exist for our entry and use or they would not exist at all. This addresses the tendency for some people to believe they cannot become what or how they want, perhaps feeling undeserving. The invitation to associate permanently into a state exists as evidenced simply by the presence of the resource states. They do not exist so we cannot operate from them. Rather, they exist so we can associate into them for some constructive purpose.

> The word universe is an interesting word, one verse with an infinite number of variations within the theme. Artists, whether visual, auditory, gustatory or otherwise, remind us of how well the universe fits together by showing different sounds, flavors, shapes or colors harmoniously and naturally interacting.
>
> Even movement, animate or inanimate, can remind us of the universal interacting of all elements. It just goes to show you. We feel comforted, reassured, safe and inspired by their message no matter the form of their communicating. No risk you know?
>
> And you want to exemplify one certain kind of variation within the infinite collection? Yet you seem to believe you

cannot. But how did you know the certain way exists? Didn't you imagine it, which means it exists or you could not have imagined it? And to imagine it didn't you have to actually go to it. Otherwise you could not describe it or know it.

By the way, how will you know you are there? Answering this question requires you go there, doesn't it? Why not stay? So you know the place and you know the way, then the issue becomes why can't you yet stay. Not quite fully believing you can stay or is it doubt you can go at all? Well, the doubt leaves when you enter, as you have already experienced. They are mutually exclusive.

The more you enter the less the doubt, no doubt, certain. And you may wonder if it is OK for you to go and stay. If you enter it means the state exists and it is there for you. What being created these places? Nothing exists for no reason and not utilizing these places by design goes against the design. So as you enter this state by the creator, let the most uncertain part go first as to not be left behind. This reluctance is just inverted eagerness, isn't it? Feel this propel you toward this, and how.

And you may also wonder, when you get it will it leave you? Look around and note what is stationary and receptive, it's your move. Not trusting only deceives your self. The proof is in the putting. Now you know all of you desires going to places you have not gone to before but want to. And these places exist so you can go there. Now, you already know this. How will this new way alter the way you do? By design.

Chapter Eight
Language Patterns Addressing States of Mind-Emotion

We know of several reasons for constructing language patterns addressing states of mind-emotion. The state of mind-emotion a person occupies at any given time may very well exert more influence on the individual than any other element. These other influential elements include thoughts, behaviors and environmental stimuli. Whatever a person thinks or displays behaviorally seems to stem from his state of mind-emotion.

My belief is that states are made up of thoughts, behaviors and stimuli sensed in the environment. A person considers these elements and then generates a state, a sort of conclusion, depending on her particular Meta-programs. The influence of these non-state elements is that they can, by changing, exert an influence on a state and actually change the state through dissonance reduction. A shy (state) person may sustain the state by a belief that if she asserts herself she'll face rejection by others. But one day she asserts herself (behavioral change) and this brings approval by others. Then the previous belief about others may be changed. But primarily the state has the most influence in a person's life because it seems to direct the person's perception-behavior.

The state determines the thoughts, emotions and behavior of the person. By thoughts, we refer to the awareness of and identifying of information before actually assembling them into a conclusion. This is much like sensation without perception. The conclusion, or meaning-making that comes with perception, equates to a belief and exerts its own significant influence. Because beliefs exert their own distinct influence, we included earlier a separate section devoted to hypnotic language and beliefs (chapter 4).

States of mind-emotion range from joy to curiosity to despair to exhilaration and include many more. You can also move to a Meta-state position as described by Hall (1996). This position results in states of mind-emotion about previous states of mind-emotion. As a result, these states modify the prior states. In this way you can experience curiosity about your anger. As a result, you can move a person to more constructive responses, instead of just experiencing anger, guilt or righteousness about your anger. Meta-states open up the person to broader awareness and therefore, more choices and possibilities. The more Meta-state levels you put on the ladder, the higher functioning level available for the individual.

Meta-states open up the person to broader awareness and therefore, more choices and possibilities. The more Meta-state levels you put on the ladder, the higher functioning level available for the individual.

But people do not always use these meta-levels for constructive action. Sometimes meta-levels only intensify a limiting state and result in some self-limiting state. A person can experience anger at the primary level and then experience fear of her anger and then experience anger at the fear of the anger. This may result in self-contempt. I find that personality disordered clients seem to use meta-levels to maintain a self-limiting style. It seems as if all levels serve to maintain the dysfunction. Meta-levels can create prisons as provided by the example Bob gave at the beginning of chapter 5. At the same time, the general truth needing to be stated here is that meta-levels do at least provide an opportunity for a person to function at a higher and more effective level. Therefore, our meta-levels can both determine our hell or our heaven.

Our meta-levels can both determine our hell or our heaven.

States of mind-emotion act as filtering devices and become what we call Meta-programs in NLP, and determine what we perceive. Each state makes perceptual filters that perpetuate the status quo (Burton, 1998). Changing what we perceive may alter the state if the new perception possesses enough intensity or volume to out-weigh the current collection of evidence supporting the status quo. But changing the state of mind-emotion seems to always alter the information the individual perceives.

One of the most crucial steps in effective therapy involves helping the client move to and utilize more resourceful states of mind-emotion. Sometimes the client puts up various subtle or obvious objections to the more resourceful state, becoming reluctant to occupy or associate into the state. Other times the client finds it difficult or uncomfortable to remain in the more resourceful state.

Additionally, just helping the client expand her awareness of other states to choose from may in itself lift the client out of a stuck spot. As an analogy, the driver remembers that second gear continues existing and is available, even though she may currently be using fourth gear in her manual transmission. With this reminder, a person remembers that options exist for use in various conditions.

With the above principles and purposes in mind, the following hypnotic language patterns present themselves as methods of change-making through the use of states of mind-emotion:

Go Unconscious: *Accessing Cooperation*

This hypnotic language intervention occurred in the midst of a session with a particular client who claimed he could not stay alert. The original reason he came to counseling was for treatment of the 'feeling of depression'. During this particular session, this client reported that he felt extremely drowsy and was experiencing a great deal of difficulty paying attention to what I said.

His body language verified that he felt drowsy as he slouched in the chair with his eyes only half-open. He said that he could think of no reason for feeling so tired. He had slept well the night before and was not drowsy earlier in the session. But, as we moved into the session, he stated that he could barely pay attention to what was going on.

At first I interpreted his behavior as some sort of bid for control through resistance by claiming he was almost immune to our interaction. Whether or not this interpretation held any validity became mute. The following pattern simply utilizes what the client gave me and I reframed it into something that would result in his alliance with me regardless of how he responded.

The pattern combines reframing within a double bind process. Egocentrism, continuation as well as simplicity also figure in the process. He could not help but apply the words to himself since egocentrism makes it human nature to do so. Once started in a particular state, cooperation in this case, a person tends to remain there due to the principle of continuation. Once directly accessing his unconscious mind, he will experience the simplicity of this method and maintain it, rather than muddling through the layers of defense mechanisms or compensation.

The pattern also creates dissonance by splitting up the presentation of self into two parts—'drowsy' and 'can't pay attention'. I then made each at odds with his original presentation of being drowsy. 'Drowsy' and 'can't pay attention' now represented choices. But after the hypnotic pattern is spoken, each choice complies with the therapist's preference that he tune in to his unconscious mind or tune in more to the 'here and now' conscious interaction going on between the two of us. Either way results in a more effective interaction with the client on an unconscious level or a conscious one. The actual effect resulted in quite a deep and cooperative trance for the client who developed an effective ability to release his depression and replace it with a comforting calm and safe state.

> Roger, I know you say that you feel tired and that you can barely pay attention to what I am saying and that you feel like you might almost fall asleep. But what this really means is that your unconscious mind is in complete control as you sit there feeling drowsy. And this is a good thing because your unconscious mind can more fully hear and pay attention to what I say so that you can more fully understand and use your deepest resources to make the kind of changes that you know you want to make.

> By being so drowsy this permits more communication with your unconscious mind allowing your unconscious mind to more fully help you become how you most want to be. So I encourage you to remain sitting there with your conscious mind barely able to pay attention so that your unconscious mind can pay more attention. And then fully release any depression your conscious mind had replacing it with this deepest of relaxed and peaceful feelings that you can keep now and in the future noticing all the possibilities for feeling and using this deepest sense of relaxed and peaceful feelings.

Boring: *Shifting Away from Boring into Choice*

This pattern addresses the dynamics of boredom. The pattern highlights two perspectives. The first refers to the idea that people tend to get bored when they do not experience things in sufficient depth to notice more interesting elements. This leaves the person hopping from one shallow experience to another shallow experience.

The second dynamic comes from an experience with a client who discovered that he tended to keep working on the same tasks over and over without ever completing any of them. He did this because he believed that after he completed a task he'd be lost without direction and this would result in him becoming bored. As so often happens, the strategy used for preventing what he did not want (boredom) actually resulted in his obtaining what he did not want—boredom. So the hypnotic pattern comments on these dynamics.

I also added the 'Apply to Self' question for this particular client, 'How boring is it to keep doing the same things over and over?' But this pattern in general invites the listener to associate into the language pattern when it shifts from 'a mine' to a 'yours', playing on similarity with the word mine. Communicating with homonyms grants entry into other words of a similar sound since similar sounding words get grouped together in the mind (NLP phonological ambiguity). Accessing this group of similar sounding words then allows you to choose a similar sounding word and yet one that has a very different meaning.

Note: Here I apply boredom back on itself thus generating an NLP sleight of mouth pattern called 'Apply to Self'. (See Hall and Bodenhamer, *Mind Lines: Lines for Changing Minds*, 1997b.)

This pattern uses the current state (boredom-boring) and draws upon similarity again to access other, more resourceful uses of the same sounding word. Boring becomes a verb that invites the listener to bore more deeply into a subject to find more interesting aspects. In addition to similarity, dissonance gets created with the use of 'the idea held interest'. This phrase represents an example of syntactic ambiguity from the Milton model of language

(Chapter Nine). The 'held interest' can mean the idea is interesting or the idea itself can actively hold on to interest. The reference to 'holding interest' subtly invites the listener access to their own state of interest and allows them to hold on to it. And finally, the listener receives an invitation to fully experience, or associate into and employ new resources with the ending tag question that seeks ecological agreement.

In addition to the earlier client application, I applied this particular pattern in the case of a client who found it difficult to sustain any one interest or endeavor over a prolonged period of time. This 18-year-old male possessed many skills and talents from music to athletics along with very fine academic abilities. Once he started a variety of activities or projects, he often became bored soon after attaining an early success. It seemed the challenge disappeared after a short while. So for this client I attempted to point him in the direction of sustaining efforts in order to yield deeper and more interesting experiences.

One of this client's goals stated at the beginning of therapy included making a decision about his academic future. He could not decide whether to drop out of the private high school he attended; get his high school equivalency degree; or enroll at a public high school after sitting out this semester. This client ended up choosing to return to the private school and complete his studies to receive his diploma. He expressed much relief about this decision to follow through on his academics to completion.

> How do you know when you feel bored? No doubt you started your endeavor with best intentions and the idea held interest. And when you started the experience you found interesting things sort of like going into a mine except it is yours. You can notice how at first a few smaller gems become evident but these become dull shortly.
>
> By boring down more deeply you can find the larger more evolved gems. These gems, minerals and resources spent more time developing and you can notice their larger multi-faceted qualities, purer yet diverse, singularly and collectively. This is not boring boring, yet it bores the resources out of the depths as you feel them rise to your surface for your use, aren't they now?

Occasional Table: *Remembering States Not Being Used*

This short pattern simply asks the listener to dissociate from an unwanted, limiting state and then to search through her unconscious awareness of all that is not this unwanted state. A figure-ground reversal serves as the method of shifting awareness. Various dissociating techniques also get used and identified in the text. You can leave out the attempt at humor if you find it either not humorous for you or the client, or if is it is not your style.

The pattern aims to tune the listener into all other possibilities, restoring choice. The therapist can put at the end of the pattern whatever problem state the client is experiencing. I used depression in this case as an example. Anxiety, jealousy or any other state can be plugged in at the end. Once the client shifts out of the unwanted state, the therapist can assist her in choosing a more resourceful state.

> You, no doubt, have heard of a piece of furniture known as a table, right? Four legs and a flat top, and yet that's not a band from the fifties. [*I hope to dissociate the listener here through the use of humor.*] And you may even visualize some of the tables you have seen from your past, recalling a variety. [*Pause a few seconds to allow the client to do this visualizing if she seems to be visualizing.*]
>
> And as you do, you can probably remember the setting of these tables you see and even how you felt while you were there. [*This statement further dissociates the client from the emotional state she started with.*] And you probably have heard of a particular kind of table known as an occasional table, right?
>
> Well, hear… what I wonder. What is the table when it is not a table? If it is an occasional table, what is it when it's not a table? And now you may ask yourself and answer now, what are you when you are not depressed?

Discouragement: *Converting Disappointment into Determination*

This simple, direct and short pattern works on the dynamics of discouragement. The words present an alternative response to circumstances that often lead to a state of discouragement. Instead of producing discouragement, not reaching one's desired outcome can, as the pattern suggests, serve to fuel the fire of determination.

> Disappointments can seem like trees, small or large, watched falling in the forest. Maybe you feel grief over this loss. But consider converting all disappointments into logs fueling the purpose, making it grow stronger and brighter. As you imagine this, you can even feel the increasing warmth throughout your entire being and seeing more with this illuminating glow. You can use this now, can't you… see, feel and realize your strength increasing until…you know, don't you?

Doubt: Removing the Interference of Doubt

This hypnotic pattern addresses the dynamics of doubting. In particular, doubt related to resource states that reside within a person. Doubt dilutes the purity and strength of any state, resource or belief. Doubt prevents a person from fully associating into any state. Essentially, doubt requires a particular perspective about some information. This perspective consists of the doubter shifting back and forth between belief and disbelief but never fully embracing either position.

But doubt exists about some information so the information's existence occurs first, followed by the state of doubt. Doubt in essence says one thing may be true but again it may not be true, for something else may be true. We alternate between at least two concepts by affirming one then disaffirming it and moving our focus to the other alternative and affirming it. In essence we say, 'Maybe A is true but maybe not. Maybe B is true instead of A'. In the process, we at least momentarily say that 'A' maybe true and for that moment 'A' exists in our awareness.

Doubt in essence says one thing may be true but again it may not be true, for something else may be true.

By just acknowledging that some general information exists, doubted or not, this permits altering thoughts of doubt to acknowledging that some general information exists. Once this removal of doubt happens, the client has moved to state choice, which replaces doubt. The client can then choose how he wants to feel or think about the information. This altering of thoughts happens by reversing the time sequence of events, going back in time to before doubt. This process leaves just the information sensed. A reframe of sorts, in this pattern shifts the listener from doubt to belief that some general information exists.

This pattern also invokes confidence as an alternative state to doubt. A sort of double bind takes place by linking doubt and confidence ('Do you doubt your confidence or feel confident in your doubt?') thereby, introducing the state of confidence in as being undeniable either way the client answers. The listener's confidence also receives a wake-up call by accessing any past successes to build upon in the present and future.

Resources in the listener's secondary awareness receive a call to be remembered when the 'general outranks a specific' line invites a broadening of the listener's perspective. This also meta-states the client (Hall, 1996). The reference to 'proving' (Second paragraph), suggests utilizing more general abilities rather than getting bogged down in the specific details of a single task. With this comes a meta-stating above the one with narrower awareness. Reframing doubt to include a more resourceful meaning also relies on secondary awareness. The very first line sets a tone of confusion or dissonance (syntactic ambiguity) by referring to doubt but not specifically stating what to doubt.

The purpose of asking 'are you confident about your doubt or do you doubt your confidence' is to gain access to the state of confidence either way the listener answers. The state of confident becomes available for stepping into because the state is a part of either answer. Now he has checkmated himself. I use this sort of sleight of mouth pattern a lot on other states as well. Combine the limiting state with a rough estimate of it's inverse and pair them together. Either way, you get access to the desired state.

You know, when you think about your doubt you find that in fact you must have something to doubt. This means you must first acknowledge something may be present in order to doubt. Because the only way to doubt is to first believe because you know you do not doubt when you know something is not there. And you do not doubt when you know something is present.

Two ways to not doubt, no doubt. And when you seek to prove something you doubt you only prove you doubt that which is already present. Consider the issue of trying to prove you can succeed. [*The therapist can refer to any specific issue that the client wants to verify about himself such as being lovable or acceptable.*] Have you ever succeeded once? If the answer is yes, and you know it is, then you have proven your ability to succeed. Attempting to further prove what has already been proven only proves you doubt what you really know. So do you doubt your confidence or feel confidence in your doubt? Either way you can feel confidence, can't you?

And a general outranks a specific. Just what are you trying to prove? So doubt really means you know something is present. Since you do not doubt its presence what is it you actually feel? Perhaps just an increased desire to know more, deeply, about what you already know is present because the more deeply you feel the more clear and secure the root.

Doubt invites a closer look informing you so can better use your interest and curiosity to k-n-o-w more about what you know you already possess, don't you, feel this now and imagine the ways to use this already proven ability, that you know?

As Good As Done: *Removing Pressure to Enhance Performance with Relief*

This simple pattern first invites the listener to associate into a pressure-filled situation from his past. The listener is then asked to shift states to one of relief that normally happens when one gets close to completing a tough project. The client is then asked to imagine replacing the limiting state of feeling pressure with the resources of the state of relief. This shift of states is then Future

Paced as the listener imagines applying the state of relief to a future opportunity.

> You know how it feels when you work on a project, especially one you know is very important? You may feel a sense of pressure or urgency along with some general mental and physical tightness and gradual loss of energy. Now remember how you feel when you know you are near completion, when you are as good as done? You may feel pressure lift, replaced by relief and a return of energy and flexibility. How will it feel when you start the same project with this feeling of being as good as done? I guess you won't know until you're as good as done. And what is it like when you are as good as done with implanting this as good as done feeling in any future event?

Good Gulf: *Depression and Loss*

The contents of this pattern relate to the dynamics of depression. This pattern also addresses grief and loss as these two components often reside in, and in fact help create, depression. The use of dissonance, similarity and continuation occur several times. Dissonance and similarity occur with the reference to the two kinds of gulf-golf and the one with 'U'—you in it. The last paragraph suggests continuation.

Reference to all five senses, about one-third of the way through, brings about dissonance. But this reference to the five senses also makes for a deeper trance experience and future application (future pace) of the constructive resources. Reconciling depression or grief, with each involving a loss, comes from closing the gap or gulf left from the loss.

Depression or grief requires a specific and general component. The depression or loss involves general traits or states from the past experience or relationship. The specific portion of this recovery process involves specific opportunities available in the future to apply these formerly lost states that the client now understands as resources. They become resources because the person 'preserves' the fond memories and useful learnings gained from the former relationship. Thus, the former grief sufferer re-experiences what, in a depressed state, seemed losses but in the resourceful present and future are framed as resources. This re-experiencing, or associating into a state, fills the 'loss gulf', allowing full recovery in every sense.

You know a gulf is that space between two areas such as bodies, land, groups of people or even political stances and budding romances. And there is another kind of gulf, one with an 'O' in it instead of 'U'. You know, that golf involving fowl such as birdies and eagles.

Well, anyway, returning to the gulf with 'U' in it. I was recently talking with a friend, who was going through quite a challenge, a tough decision with two clear sides to it, yes, a gulf. The more he talked, expressing his concern, the more I listened and the more I listened the more my face began looking like his. My look clearly registered with him so I said, I can tell you see I hear you feel unsure about this dilemma. It sort of brought him to his senses. Then it also dawned on me he is going through one of those approach–avoidance conflicts, kind of like a tug-of-war with relatives pulling on each side so you don't quite know whom to root for. Good is present on both sides.

The core of the matter occurred to me. One part is general and the other specific. I mean the part we want to avoid losing is the general and the part we want to approach is specific. One is past while the other is present and future. Take for instance a job you might consider leaving. Certainly unpleasant parts lead to wanting to leave. Yet when you think about what you like, you'd miss by leaving. Then you think about what you'd gain by leaving. You find yourself experiencing the gulf.

When you are not where you don't want to be you will miss 'X'. This tells you to stay. But when you are there, staying, you will miss 'Y'. But there are several things that make staying unpleasant and these tell you to go. Further, you know of something better to go to. Reconciling comes from taking the general parts you would miss and placing them with the specific parts you will gain to make a full recovery.

This same process plays out when you grieve, then recover. You recover inside but you also recover or reclaim the best of the general traits you thought lost in the departed incorporating them into your daily life for displays of honor. Keep the best general and apply specifically here and now. Then you won't be able to miss it because it will appear right before you eyes. You even do the same when you recover lost aspects of yourself from your past, lost parts of yourself from childhood, you know. Recover the general with up-to-date fabric and use it with joy today and tomorrow.

Impulsively Foresighted: Converting Impulsiveness into Foresight

This pattern addresses two separate states, impulsive and foresight. While at first glance these two states seem opposites, this pattern seeks to merge them into a useful team. Using the energizing state of impulsive to corral energy, the pattern starts with impulsive and invites the listener to associate into the state.

For a more complete associating into the state, I lay out the dynamics of impulsiveness. I also utilize myself as the subject of the story thus decreasing potential defensiveness on the part of the client and increase receptivity in the listener (Milton model extended quotes). By using myself as the object, I deflect any resistance from the client to myself, the object of the quotes. The state of curiosity gets applied to impulsive for a more objective yet motivated consideration of impulsiveness.

Later I invite the listener to search for matching dynamics within themselves. Egocentricity will naturally lead to this applying to self within the client. Following this I suggest the listener associate into the new state and notice how he can utilize the duo of foresight and impulsive in the future.

> Just recently I was remembering an incident when I felt especially impulsive. You know the feeling, when you believe you just can't wait or do not want to wait and there is this pressing energizing feeling in you. It comes from the desire to make something important happen now, not later.
>
> Once I started thinking, really thinking about how this impulse feeling came to be, I was curious about my impulsiveness. Well, what I discovered, and you may find this true for you as well, was that my impulsiveness actually comes

out of this speed of light foresight. My impulsiveness actually stems from its inverse, foresight. This is amazing to me.

I used to think all I felt was impulsive when actually I felt foresight first. Apparently I look ahead and realize time is limited for accomplishing important tasks. Even as I recall this awareness, I feel the return of the impulse. But what makes such a modifying difference is realizing how my foresight can interact with my impulsiveness. And in fact my impulsiveness follows my foresight, so these two can work together.

Foresight can go out as a scouting expedition searching for the proper time to act. Then blending the urge to act with the awareness of timing so just the right time can be found for the best outcome. Naturally this is preceded by and depends on trusting your awareness of your foresight and impulsive parts. We might refer to this as forepulse.

As long as we are discussing pulses, allow yourself to consider the one known as compulsive that often marries obsessive to form one of those hyphenated names, obsessive-compulsive. From what I can tell, and I'm telling all that I know, this obsessive-compulsive routine stems from short-sighted persistence, like a headlight pointing down at the ground immediately in front instead of showing the way a way off in the distance to ingest and accommodate moving toward the lighted goal. It never reaches the conclusion because it misses key ingredients.

But the belief that ingredients and desired outcome are all inclusive in the present causes pointless persistence in going over the same old ground driven by the same old belief. It is like cookie dough being made and the raw dough is arranged on a sheet over and over but not one is placed in the oven for finishing. The hunger accumulates and only results in faster cookie forming but still no baking. What's missing?

The general process is a very good one in that it uses determination to pursue what it most desires. The only flaw in the system is where the work is being done which results in it never being done.

The o-c, if you will, mistakenly believes the solution is in the details at hand but the real solution and satisfying outcome involves a bigger picture with bigger parts stretching out over a longer span of time. A big picture trying to fit into a small frame and it's not accommodating. No wonder you feel tight.

This dogged persistence, like a hound on the trail, will serve the cause well and will cause the solution to be realized in the future over time, including the formerly missing, now found in the future. Do not open 'til...you know... the right time. Let the awareness of needed parts determine where to search not just time or location.

The latter causes a repeating loop, loop that takes on dizzying proportions. The former, raised and forward aiming, permits forward movement to the fulfilling goal. So when the couple, obsessive—compulsive, come to visit, and they're usually early, just look up and apply their eagerness in the present to the future. While not ill they will make for good patience, just wait and see for yourself.

Persistence Resistance: Overcoming Procrastination

Here, the emphasis is placed on the dynamics of procrastinating, the positive purpose of this and then converting procrastination into motivating action. At times procrastination may involve a shortsighted strategy designed to avoid a negative outcome or loss of control. This concern is addressed by pointing out that the likely result of procrastinating will be the very outcome the client is attempting to avoid, thus encouraging a change of choice.

> **'How will your method of preventing a bad outcome by choosing a bad outcome accomplish your goal?'**

The last sentence summarizes the principle at work here by asking, 'How will your method of preventing a bad outcome by choosing a bad outcome accomplish your goal?' Dissonance reduction drive makes this a change-compelling tactic. Aligning desired outcome with chosen strategy permits continuation and similarity to work effectively.

213

Procrastinating is an incessant effort at making no effort. It only puts off relief. But you cannot not persist. Persistence transforms the foreign into the familiar. Just how do you know? Choose what you want to become familiar with. And you know of course, you cannot not choose either. Any way you go is with persistence, much like your shadow, it follows up your every move.

Now you may try outsmarting the whole insurrection by repeatedly changing direction so that you do not persist at any one connection. But what do you do then with persistence? [*I use a double question here utilizing the similarities concept with the concept-word 'persistence.' Not only will you use it to incessantly shift, but then, what else can you do with the quality known as 'persistence'?*] Persistence resistance makes a dam. Do you want a flood or a stream? One you can control while the other goes to the extreme. How will not taking action keep you from falling short of your goal?

Quite a Flap: Accessing Assertiveness

I address the state of assertiveness in this pattern. The state and dynamics of assertiveness get explained in this story with reference to the usefulness of assertiveness for independent well-being. Within the story, recruiting the state of 'open to new information', or learning, provides an assisting device for acquiring assertiveness. This learning state then acts as a device encouraging the listener to associate into assertiveness thus integrating the state within the self.

By learning I don't just mean that the client takes in one-dimensional information but that they consider all the possibilities about the new information. The story progresses from a negative scenario, in the absence of assertiveness, to a positive outcome involving freedom by utilizing assertiveness. This provides a two-way motivation. Without assertiveness, self-limitations take over, making this an outcome to avoid. While with assertiveness, the sky becomes the limit.

This story may be more suited to children but could also be presented to adults. With adults, the therapist may introduce the story as being more for children but set a frame that just maybe the adult client could appreciate the intent of the story as well. The hypnotherapist may wish to say to an adult, 'You know, this story I want to tell you is really designed for children. But maybe you can listen to it and still find something useful in it, especially if you listen to it like a child would, you know?' This sort of introduction acknowledges the adult mentality but also accesses the child mentality within the adult. And, it is this child mentality that needs most to hear the story since the child mentality is where the limitations reside.

> This is a story about a bird. This bird's name is Hue. Hue grew up healthy and happy and knows how to fly very well. He can go fast, slow, coast or soar and even fly low to the ground. He is a very wise bird and really likes learning a lot.
>
> Hue has this very interesting and unusual style about him. When he is scared his wings do not flap. But, whenever he gets mad his wings begin flapping. So you can just picture this, when he feels angry and starts talking about it, his wings flap. The more he feels angry, the more and faster his wings flap.
>
> Also, Hue has another amazing way about him that makes his wings flap. Whenever he is learning something his wings start flapping. The more he is learning and understanding the more his wings flap. When he is learning, his mind is just going a hundred miles-an-hour thinking about the new information and processing it deeply. His wings just reflect what his mind is doing.
>
> Why one day he learned so much his wings moved like a humming bird's. Now these are not the only times Hue flaps his wings. He can also just decide to flap his wings and he does, then he flies.
>
> One day while out flying, and Hue was not angry or learning anything new in particular, a storm began building and it got very windy. Hue knew the rain would soon fall and flying would be more difficult. So Hue decided to fly home before the weather got too nasty. Well the storm moved in faster than expected. The wind blew and the rain came down very hard. Flapping furiously Hue tried steering himself toward his home. He was sort of scared and this made flapping more difficult but he kept trying hard to keep his wings flapping in

the stiff breeze. Suddenly a gust of wind burst over him sending him crashing to the ground. Hue landed on one of his wings and let out a loud 'OUCH!' Now he was scared and hurt.

He could not move his wing that hurt and his fear made his wings still anyway. What would he do? Well fortunately, another bird living nearby saw the whole thing and hopped over to where Hue was huddled. This bird lived in a house in the bushes near the ground level as some birds do. This bird's name is Harper.

Well Harper offered Hue a place to come in from the storm. Hue was in no place to refuse so he hopped along behind Harper to his nest in the thick bushes. No doubt this nest was warmer and drier and it sure felt safer. There was plenty of room for each to rest comfortably. Harper thought it was best for Hue to stay for awhile until he got to feeling better. After all, Hue couldn't move his injured wing and how could he possibly fly?

Harper helped Hue and provided a safe place from the storm and for Hue to mend his injured wing. Hue felt very grateful and settled in for recovery. The storm clouds gradually gave way to thinner and thinner, lighter and lighter clouds until the sunshine pushed through. This certainly felt welcome as they prepared for the coming evening.

The new day followed nightfall but Hue's wing still felt painful and could not move comfortably so he stayed on. Several days came and went. Harper continued tending Hue. Harper insisted Hue not even lift his wing, let alone try to fly. Days piled up of limited movement and restriction with the intention of healing.

Harper continued instructing Hue to be still and not move or use his injured wing. Hue felt growing curiosity about the progress of his wing's healing. Restless, Hue began shifting back and forth within the nest but just could no longer find a comfortable spot. He longed to fly again. All the while Harper continued caretaking. Harper simply would not permit Hue to use his injured wing and insisted on providing for Hue.

Now friction began between the two, as Hue grew increasingly curious and even eager to test out his wing. After all, several weeks have passed. A sort of tug-of-war developed, slowly and gently at first but more and more the two disagreed out in the open. Harper felt sure that Hue's wing was still not ready for flight while Hue felt he needed to know this for sure. The only way to really know is to do it, thought Hue.

Things we do not do that we know we need to do have a way of reminding us they are not done. This is the case with Hue. He knew he simply must use his wing and fly. Yet this still had not happened. One day, Hue reached the limit of waiting. He and Harper had it out. All the stored energy Hue kept suddenly spilled out. Hue got angry while telling Harper it was time to fly.

While Harper and Hue got more and more angry, Hue's wings just started flapping as they do when he gets mad. At first Hue did not notice, habits you know, but then Hue could tell he was flapping and then he began realizing, learning you know, which only made his wings flap faster and harder until Hue lifted off the ground. No longer angry, Hue continued realizing and learning, now rising above Harper.

The more Hue made sense of the situation the more it fueled his flapping. Soon Hue rose higher and higher to realize he knew he could now fly just fine. He left his anger behind and flew off knowing. Home is a great place to be, thought Hue, as he made himself comfortable in his favorite place, just the way he chooses.

See What You Think: Shifting from Anxiety Back to Choice

The hypnotic language pattern here specifically addresses anxiety, but generally addresses the principle involved when the brain envisions and/or pursues an outcome. Much dissonance (repeated reference 'to think' and 'to see' in differing orders) and similarity ('piece-peace', 'there as well') as well as continuation play throughout the pattern. The successive use of the phrases 'you know' as well as the successive use of 'you see' create dissociation in the listener. Once dissociated from an old, limiting state, the client can then associate into a more resourceful state. The finishing ambiguous reference to 'right, now' refers to the described strategy being the right choice 'now' and putting the strategy into use 'right now.'

> **Once dissociated from an old, limiting state, the client can then associate into a more resourceful state.**

So you say you feel anxious in this certain situation. [*The therapist can specify the situation.*] Well take a moment and think about the circumstance leading to your anxiety... See what you think... and then think what you see. In fact, this is the real problem you know, thinking what you see, you see, the pieces you fear and then think of the fear that causes no peace. When there is no piece, p-i-e-c-e, you experience only the void or, deeper, place of pure potentiality and we always see what we think and think what we see so decide what you most want to see n-o-w, because you know it is there as well.

Allow yourself to think what you want to, see? So now you see what you know you want and think what you know you want, you know this... will naturally cause you to be and act the way you think you want to be, n-o-w, isn't it? I dare not say this will transform into a most useful universal strategy for you, so see what you think and think what you see deciding what you want, n-o-w including how this feels, right, now.

Serve it Up: Developing Foresight, Patience and Flexibility

This story involves needs—meeting of needs and how a person can balance needs with effectively satisfying the needs. Overcoming impulsiveness to develop foresight and other ingredients necessary to satisfy needs is a recurrent theme throughout the story. The story plays to most of the five senses to enrich the awareness and deepen the trance-involvement of the listener. Since states drive behavior, the story attempts to shift the client from states that lead to undesirable outcomes to states that lead to desirable outcomes.

If a state can become associated with the desired outcome (whenever I trust myself I end up with good results and then I feel good) then the goal becomes maintaining or attaining the state (trust of self) because it brings the person what he wants. The consequences of using the state simply reinforce further use. And, any outcome not consistent with the resource state will be avoided. For example, the thought, 'I got in trouble because I said "yes" to someone when my gut told me to say "no". Next time I will trust my gut instinct' will be avoided in favor of outcomes consistent with the positive state. The result is first associating into the resource-state and then deciding what behavior is best.

> This story concerns three cooks. They feel concerned because each is hungry and wants to eat. They feel that stirring hunger in their stomach. You know the one that makes your stomach growl. Maybe it's angry over impatience over eager, almost like eggs over easy or hard but different.
>
> These three cooks live in different homes in different parts of the same town and are all related. Coming from the same family and being raised together results in their being pretty similar in preference and taste. This particular day each feels hungry at about the same time and decides to take care of this need by cooking their favorite dish. It so happens that each of them have the same favorite dish.
>
> They know the dish requires certain ingredients in order to turn it into what they most like. Each cook gathers the ingredients and prepares them the same, in just the right manner. This particular favorite is a casserole. Once the ingredients get combined in their proper amount, the whole collection gets placed in the oven at a certain temperature for a certain amount of time. But on this day the hunger of the three is quite strong and compelling. How will they negotiate the time between want and fulfillment to end up with what they desire?
>
> Three strategies take action. The first cook, knowing the dish needs one hour to cook fully at a certain temperature, decides to try intervening in the natural course of events by turning up the temperature. If the casserole needs one hour at this temperature then if the temperature is turned up to almost twice as high it will be done in about half the time. This seemed to make logical sense just based on simple math, ignoring other elements.
>
> So the first cook turned up the temperature as high as the oven would go and set the timer for just a half-hour. At precisely one half-hour later the cook removed the dish from the oven placing it on the top of the stove for examination.

Whew, what a sight! Having never checked on the cooking process at any point during the half-hour, no adjustments could be made because there was no progress to consider. Looking at the casserole, it sort of evolved in a layered fashion in thirds. The top layer was burned to a brittle crispiness. Digging down a little further, a layer of 'done just right' was found but it only took up about one-third of the whole casserole. The bottom third was still raw. Not being much of an archeology fan this dig held little appeal. The most this cook could do was pick around and eat parts of the middle layer after peeling away the other layers. At best this became an appetizer leaving the cook dissatisfied and still hungry.

The second cook was equally hungry and equally wondering how to take care of the hunger faster. Once the dish was prepared and placed in the oven, the watching and waiting began. During this period the overriding driving force and focus was tuning into the hunger and letting it call the shots. It was a one-track sensation bent on filling its need with nothing else considered. Tuning in to the hunger and considering only its need left little awareness of other options. This led to manipulating the only variable noticed—time. It was time to eat.

Figuring the casserole would be alright if only half cooked, how much did it really need the whole hour, the cook pulled it from the oven when the hunger just would not wait any longer. Pulling the rather loose, soupy concoction from the oven led to a deep sinking feeling. But this feeling could be ignored in the name of need. It's odd how we can ignore what we fully know when all we know is our need. It's even more interesting how you can forget how useful more information can be for more fully satisfying your need for more information to satisfy your need in whole, provided what you really most deeply want is really the most deeply satisfying feeling that you know how this feels when you more fully and deeply meet this need. How else does it work best?

So this cook began consuming the half-cooked casserole as fast as could be. It was not long before stomach pain began to override the hunger and shut off the formerly all-consuming need. Now the interest in eating totally stopped, taken over by the need to stop the pain in the pit of his stomach. No more could be eaten. While hunger was not satisfied eating more would only increase the pain. Deeply frustrated the cook paused and simply sat down, too late to wait now.

The third cook took the same ingredients and preparations combining them into the same casserole. The oven was hot for baking. And the timer was set as the cook remembered what proper timing brings. You know the correct temperature lessens the possibility of burning, actually preventing it. Sufficient cooking time permits all the parts of the casserole to fully mature, so to speak, cooking all the way from the top down to the bottom and all points in between, consistent consistency.

The best cook also uses all senses. They know when the smell means it's getting close to being done. Also they know when and what to look for when peeking at the dish while it's in progress. It even sounds a certain way as it gets closer to being done. And perhaps most importantly the best cooks know when to use a probe, going deep into the casserole and get a feel for how closely it matches the eventual finished product.

It is almost like converting just an idea into action. It starts raw but evolves into something that takes form and sub-stance that satisfies needs, well done. The cook remained determined to produce a dish resembling the picture in the cookbook that was full of recipes for satisfying meals. Just pull up the one that most appeals and follow the known instructions. They have already been tried and tested true. That is what produced the picture, it is already ready.

It's sort of like planting a tree. Before you plant you need to imagine the tree fully mature. Then choose the place best accommodating its eventual size. This is slightly different than choosing shoes while we are growing. Then we need to fit our foot for how it is, not how it will be, because then the shoe would not fit now.

Each cook determines his or her favorite recipe for satisfying hunger at the time. Maybe the one appealing is a particular ingredient or perhaps it is a collection of ingredients and their interacting that brings most satisfaction. Maybe it's a sauce or a spice or perhaps the blending of that fits like the dovetail. This particular cook just pictures what is most desired and then follows the recipe to produce.

Vanishing: Leaving Outdated States to Use New Ones

The message within this story relates to how people live by old familiar and familial ways. We each tend to repeat patterns that were present in our home during our childhood, unless we consciously intervene. The tendency often results in utilizing outdated or unsuitable resources for present day challenges.

Another level of dynamics within this story involves an internal relationship within the individual and the 'parts' of self. Often the outward display of emotion, behavior or voiced thoughts results from a power behind the scene that orchestrates the surface display. You may call this his belief and a person's belief shapes his reality. If the power behind the throne (beliefs), so to speak, is not amended then the surface collection of thoughts, emotion and behaviors is unlikely to change.

> **By reaching the belief system and communicating new information, the belief's foundation is updated, and then new behavior comes in to being.**

This tale then addresses the relationship between beliefs and behavior. The story focuses on the practical aspect of desired outcomes. If a chosen strategy brings undesired results then it becomes time to change the strategy. Perhaps the belief system in place makes for the undesired outcome. In this case it becomes time to alter the beliefs. By reaching the belief system and communicating new information, the belief's foundation is updated, and then new behavior comes in to being.

> This is a story about a man from the northern European country of Van. This makes him Vanish. It also makes the language he speaks Vanish. His lifestyle is Vanishing. He carries a name common to his home country. He is known as E'ven. Others in his home country could understand him and communicate effectively. However, problems appear when he leaves his home country of Van to find a better life.
>
> Since nobody else he encounters is Vanish he experiences much confusion and frustration in his efforts to communicate

with those who are not Vanish. Others could not make sense of his Vanishing ways. Numerous varied attempts are made but to no avail. This Vanishing man and his Vanish words fall on blind eyes and deaf ears.

All the formerly highly effective ways of the Vanish lifestyle only compound the problems. These ways all work so well in his homeland. Now these ways leave him confused and doubtful. Vanishing seems to work well back home but—come to think of it—he really just learned how to negotiate with the circumstances. He left Van because he was not happy and wants to be. But he is not happy now either. How perplexing all this all is to E'ven.

Compounding the problem is his sense of guilt for even questioning his Vanishing ways. The country has standing orders for anyone leaving Van to continue speaking Vanish and living the Vanish ways. It is supposed to reflect well on the small, tightly knit country to uphold their customs and display them to outsiders. All E'ven ever experiences from living his home customs is indifference from others, if not, downright rejection.

On one particular day, E'ven meets a man who could tell he is quite distressed. This stranger quickly becomes a compassionate friend. He takes the time to understand and decode E'ven's communication. The compassionate stranger even learns to speak Vanish. The purpose in doing so is to travel to Van.

This is done in order to explain to the leader of the Vanish life outside Van and ask the leader to permit changing the lifestyle for those traveling outside Van. It only makes good sense. Alter behavior to fit the circumstance. This need is easily confirmed by the response that is received by E'ven. The compassionate one goes on to explain that for effective living outside Van, changes must come.

Conditions in other lands differ and adjustments permit achieving the outcomes desired. New situations call for new and different choices and responses. This will lead to people from Van really making favorable impressions on others because of their effective adapting to the circumstances.

Thoroughly impressed by the reasoning of the compassionate one, the leader of the Vanish decides to change the rules of behavior. The Vanish no longer have to speak Vanish or live Vanishing ways outside the country. They are free to adapt to the environment and conditions of wherever they live. Vanish living outside Van now seek what works to create desired outcomes and lead them to satisfaction and fulfillment.

It turns out that E'ven settles in a country known as Fin. Do not confuse this with the fine, industrious, determined and fun-loving people of Finland. However, the people of Fin are also known as Finish. Now E'ven lives the life of the Finish, speaks Finish and he believes he is Finish. E'ven certainly feels very Finish now.

It's Not Worth Feeling Guilty: Moving Past Guilt to *Positive Action*

> **It seems that for guilt to exist a person must disconnect from a sense of self-worth.**

The narrative below addresses the dynamics of guilt. By guilt, I mean self-attacks in which the person devalues herself. Regret and remorse exist as states about a behavior or lack thereof. But guilt takes this a step further to include an attack on self. It seems that for guilt to exist a person must disconnect from a sense of self-worth. Because the supposed offender feels guilt over an action or lack of action, she disconnects from positive worth. She does this believing she does not deserve the resources that positive self-worth bring. Yet, worth awareness contains the necessary resources for resolving the concern.

Guilt locks us out of the house without a key. All of our resources, however, reside within the house. Once returning to awareness of inherent worth, a person finds an absence of guilt and a natural response set aimed at rectifying the undesirable act. Within this pattern the listener receives an invitation to experience a deeper and more spiritual awareness of eternal worth and the resources this provides. The title itself contains the double message that conveys this principle.

So you believe you offended someone or didn't defend someone? And now how will you fend off guilt? What will allow you to send guilt away and feel good about this putting an end to, saying amen to? Do you find guilt revolves around a belief that you did not live up to your values? Beneath this is it that you then question your worth for not doing so?

As best as I can tell, and you know asbestos is a known health hazard, guilt is the last link in a chain preceded by doubting self-worth. You cannot experience guilt without first doubting. This doubt applied to self-worth allows guilt to creep in through the crack in the door that is ajar. Doubt seems a wedge driven between our self and our awareness of worth. It separates us from our worth and may then result in some separation anxiety you know.

But looking back don't you have to have experienced something in order to doubt it? Otherwise you have nothing to doubt but what you imagine. Now don't you imagine this is true? Then isn't it true that you already have worth but just doubt your right to regain it? Perhaps then, you feel guilty about your worth. But I ask you, is worth based on what you do, your actions only? Do not your actions spring from some source or reservoir? From where does the wherewithal to act come? This place of action origin, is this truly your worth?

So then actions do not make your worth but they come from this constant pool of worth within. Do you only feel worth when displaying this pool or can the consistent awareness of this pool provide the source that is the source? Does the vehicle constantly have to go full speed, to verify it is worthy? This only verifies doubt, not trust.

Doubt only proves we doubt what already exists. Continuing from here, what is the source of your source? Your reservoir results from actions of another just as your actions spring from your source. Trace this back to know your worth originates from the great spring of all waters and infinitely emits to remove limits freeing the fountain to flow out naturally. This is worth... knowing... this... now what will you choose to d-o.

[*Note*: The hypnotherapist may choose to add the following conclusion designed to move the client from 'all-or-nothing' style of thinking to a higher level of thinking, which provides for more choice and flexibility]

Now there is such a thing as o-d, but this is different than d-o. You can o-d on d-o ing. And I sure would recommend against d-o ing o-d ing. So where is the balance between o-d ing d-o ing and d-o ing o-d ing? It may seem o-d-d.

What Will You Wear it With? Freedom to Choose Any Desired State

This collection of words concerns utilizing various states that proved useful in the past but may now lie in forgotten places within the individual. The early portion of the pattern moves the listener to dissociate from a particular state and then associate him to an awareness of 'vacancy', which theoretically will make any state available.

Making use of similarity (hear–here, 'innocence in a sense' and new–knew—phonological ambiguity) and continuation allows shifting states and future orientation for use of the states. The second half of the pattern essentially takes the listener through the process of associating into a recovered state that first provides examples and then points the user towards the future for a continuation of the skill.

What if one of your five, primary senses was not functional? What if you could not hear here or anywhere for that matter? All the words in the English language and every other language would just pass by your ears, unnoticed like a tape recorder without a tape. Yet all of those words continue existing and even new ones come into existence.

And imagine that all of a sudden you became able to hear here and everywhere. Each and every word would be totally new to your ears, innocence in a sense. Yet they had long existed before you heard. It is quite exciting when you discover something new and even exciting when you discover something just new to you or something you just knew.

This is like looking into or walking more deeply into your closet of clothes and suddenly noticing an article you remember being there. Maybe you forgot for a long time and finding the once new, formerly forgotten article sort of makes it renew. You may remember where you bought it and when, suddenly feeling transported back to the store again right there in your own closet.

Usually when you find this piece you become eager to wear it and show your self and others. You try it on and notice how it feels and fits. Perhaps you already have other articles going with it and when you wear it you wear it with pride or joy or eagerness. I wonder what pieces you forgot ... you possess ... reclaiming ... renewing ... what will you wear them with?

Camping Dogs: Getting Unstuck from Resentment

This extended story involves several principles. The general theme relates to recognizing choice and foresight applied to states, behaviors and desired outcomes. Shifting the state of the listener in the process of the story also happens early through reference to removing the underlying obstacles that can impede the natural flow of water, or self in this symbolic case.

States and suggestions to implement them come in the form of the general use of flexibility, foresight and clarity of purpose through the story in a big picture perspective. Due to naturally existing egocentricity the listener will apply these traits to himself. The details simply deepen the trance by composing a more full, rich story within which the listener can more deeply emerge.

I told this true story to a female client who came in for counseling due to conflicts in her relationship with her mother. This 45-year-old client harbored huge, self-limiting loads of anger and bitterness toward her controlling mother. These thoughts, emotions and behaviors created a very self-detrimental cluster. Rather than accessing effective states of mind-emotion she accessed unproductive, limiting states. She then attributed these states to her mother and only fed her bitterness and resentment that much more fuel. Even when her mother made no attempt to intervene or interfere in her daughter's life, the client would generate imaginary thoughts for her mother and thus perpetuate the pattern, on her own. This client seemed obsessed with her mother and dwelled on past supposed injustices done to her by her.

The story emphasizes the waste of energy that harboring resentment causes and offers an alternative—to get on with life as desired resources and experiences are readily available. Once this client heard the story and the various embedded suggestions about her strategies for living, she began shifting her style. She made significant progress in disconnecting from the influence of her mother and began feeling satisfaction at determining her own thoughts, emotions and behaviors more in line with what she truly desired.

The story also provided a quick reference point which served as a gentle but clear reminder if she reverted back to her old ways. I would simply state to the client that she was barking while another bowl of food remained available or that she needed to stop barking and satisfy her hunger. She always responded with a smile that let me know the message from the original story became refreshed and applied.

> This is a true story that takes place far off in the wilderness at a campground. This is a public campground with the campsites widely spread through the woods across many acres. The only way to reach the campsites is to park your car in the car lot and then walk for a mile or more to a campsite. Many of the campsites nestle themselves along the banks of a wide and long flowing river.
>
> This story involves several people and several dogs. Three different campers with three separate tents camp together at the same site. One camper brings his two dogs. Another camper brings his dog. These three dogs all come from the same litter, two males and a female. One of the males is totally deaf. His name is Harpo and he belongs to one of the campers. The other male's name is Foster, while the female's name is Jillaroo.
>
> These two dogs belong to one of the other campers. The dogs are of a breed known as Australian Cattle Dogs or Blue Heelers. They are referred to as Blue Heelers not because they can heal the blues but because their fur gives off a blue hue, if you can picture this. The heeler part comes from their style of herding cattle. They nip at the heels of the cattle to steer them. The latter two dog's names, Foster and Jillaroo, borrow terms related to Australian life, a beer and slang for a female ranch hand.

The three campers and three dogs set up camp along the banks of this well known river that spans two states. The river possesses much character and contains several sections of rapids. You know rapids, the sections of the water that move very fast and make fairly loud noise that you can even hear off from the distance. Did you know these rapids, and any rapids, actually result from large collections of stones or boulders that lay beneath the surface of the water? This makes for more shallow and faster flowing water.

Funny how when something significant sits below the surface you can always tell where, just because it causes so much noise and forces faster movement as the water works around and over the obstacle. It impedes the flow you know?

This contrasts greatly with the slow moving and quiet stretches of water where nothing but smooth terrain rests deeply below. Imagine in the rapids section, after removing the large obstructions, freeing space to make it much deeper, how the water will feel and flow, smooth, serene, quiet and muuuch deeper. In fact, the bigger the chunk removed, the deeper the water, you know? And just how do you imagine the riverbed feels when such a big load is lifted?

Now, after setting up camp it becomes time for the dogs to eat. The one dog, Harpo and its owner, brought a bowl and food for Harpo. The other owner and his two dogs, Foster and Jillaroo, brought one bowl. These two dogs were used to eating out of the same bowl since they were brought home together at six weeks of age.

For the sake of organization, the two bowls for the three dogs are placed side-by-side and filled with dry food. Foster naturally moves to begin eating from his familiar bowl. As Foster begins eating, Harpo walks over and also begins eating from the same bowl. This new team arrangement completely throws Jillaroo off her routine.

Foster and Harpo are eating from the same bowl, hers of all things, while the second full bowl of food remains untouched. Jillaroo is a creature of habit and wants what she believes is her rightful place eating along side Foster. In order to make room for herself she begins barking at Harpo. Her request falls on deaf ears, literally. Jillaroo keeps on barking, increasing the intensity now. Foster happily continues filling his stomach from his bowl. Harpo, totally oblivious to Jillaroo, just keeps on munching in what must be to him, absolute silence. Jillaroo jockeys for different positions, closer, beside and across from but to no avail.

The two diners are nearly finished now with the whole bowl of food, while the other one remains untouched and full. Jillaroo barks incessantly and makes all kinds of motions, back and forth, kicking up dirt and aiming her snout, as if a gun, at Harpo. Nothing distracts the pair.

By now Foster and Harpo finish the entire bowl of food to the background sounds of incessant barking. And what do dogs do after they eat? They find a comfortable place to stretch out and nap. This is just what Foster and Harpo do, with Jillaroo following close behind maintaining a most amazing stream of dog cuss words, aka, barking to us humans. The two dogs that have full stomachs lay down and arrange themselves just so, closing their eyes. Jillaroo must be wondering why Harpo never pays any attention to her threats. But nonetheless, Harpo easily slips off to sleep in his silent world. Jillaroo, persistent as ever, just keeps on barking with her stomach empty. And you may wonder just how Foster managed to drift off to sleep so easily. Well, he maintained sole focus on his deeply satisfying full feeling.

Chapter Nine

The Milton Model of Language*

(*Edited from *The User's Manual for the Brain*, 1999, Bodenhamer & Hall)

> A hypnotist hypnotizes by... *saying words.*
> Pretty incredible, wouldn't you say?

What does the hypnotist do in order to hypnotize someone? When we boil it down to the basics, what do we have? What medium does a hypnotist use to affect the mind-emotions, bodies and nervous systems of those who cooperate with the process? He *simply says words.* Think about that. A hypnotist hypnotizes by... *saying words.* Pretty incredible, wouldn't you say? *'Just saying words'.* So how does that work? *How* can the saying of words 'hypnotize?'

'Hypnosis' refers to a natural process of consciousness that occurs everyday to everybody. Whenever consciousness ceases to see, hear and feel what exists immediately present in our external environment, we have 'tranced' (transitioned) out and gone somewhere else, into some internal, trance-like state. We may be 'thinking deeply', concentrating on something important, just relaxing our mind, meditating, praying, 'not thinking of anything in particular', daydreaming, etc. We may have gone inside our mind to create a vision of what we want to accomplish sometime in the future.

The fact that we seldom label such states as 'hypnotic' only serves to blind us to the regularity and commonality of this experience. It also blinds us to how easily and quickly we go in and out of altered states. What kind of a trance are you in now? What kind of trance were you in 30 minutes ago? When someone speaks to you, your brain picks up on the sound waves and at least for a brief moment, you will 'go inside'. Now, based on the structure of the words she gives you and your response to them, you will, at least for a moment, go into a trance as you 'go inside' to process what she has just spoken to you.

> **The meaning** of 'hypnosis' refers to a 'sleep-like state'
> of an intense and strong inward focus created
> primarily by trance inducing words. These words send
> us inward so that we go on a TDS (transderivational
> search) for meaning.

The meaning of 'hypnosis' refers to a 'sleep-like state' of an intense and strong inward focus created primarily by trance-inducing words. These words send us inward so that we go on a TDS (transderivational search) for meaning. Thus the power of words ultimately (and only) arises from the *reference of meaning* that we give them. We do this by 'going inward' to our internal 'library of references' that we have built up over the years in our 'memory' files where we code our understandings, values, beliefs, etc. All of this simply describes one of the powers within personality—the power to attribute meaning to things and to have an internal world.

Consider the hypnotic effects of stories and metaphors. A therapist who uses therapeutic metaphors designs them to have an isomorphic (similar) structure to the client's experience. Because of the similarity, her unconscious mind can interpret the metaphor in relation to her own needs. The client will take what she hears and represent it in terms of her own experience.

I (BB) understand that Erickson primarily used metaphor in his later years as a means of doing hypnosis. He did this for good reason. He learned through years of experience that by just 'speaking a metaphor' it would create a desire in the listener's mind to 'go inside' and put meaning to the story and to the character and incidents within the story. Metaphor provides a powerful means of doing hypnosis as the metaphors of John Burton in this book so richly reveal. And, how does one deliver a metaphor? With words of course.

> **Like metaphors, hypnotic language functions
> symbolically, as does all language.**
> Since all language functions symbolically, we can use
> language to 'create' images and meanings inside the
> head of the listener.

Like metaphors, hypnotic language functions symbolically, as does all language. The word meanings we give our experiences are just words that to us symbolize what we experience both in our external and internal worlds. Since all language functions symbolically, we can use language to 'create' images and meanings inside the head of the listener. In doing this, we are to one degree or the other 'hypnotizing' them. Our words cause them to 'go inside' and process what we have just said. This every day occurrence gives hypnosis its power—when we speak to someone and the sound waves from our mouth bounces off their eardrums, their brain must do something with that experience.

The skilled hypnotist knows how to utilize this natural phenomenon to drive the internal representations of the listener. And, of vital importance, the co-founders of NLP 'codified' the language of the great hypnotherapist Milton Erickson. In doing this, they have provided us with the structure of his language so we can duplicate that structure and re-create his genius. This 'codifying' began with the Meta-model of language and from that the Milton model of language. I will give you a summary of these models in this chapter.

The Meta-Model of Language

When we 'think' we use the representational system (rep system) of the senses: visual, auditory, kinesthetic, olfactory and gustatory (VAKOG). This enables us to *present* to ourselves *again* ('re-presentation') information that we originally saw, heard, felt, smelled, or tasted. As we use our senses we also *code those understandings in words*. Thus we can represent a pleasant summer day at the beach by using the specific sights, sounds, sensations and smells of that experience or we can use an even more short-cut system, we can say 'relaxing day at the beach'.

The words function within us as *a symbol* of the sensory representations, and those sensory representations function as a symbol of the actual experience. Thus, if we begin with the experience (the territory), our VAK representations operate as a neurological 'map' of the experience. Then our sensory-based words ('pleasant day at the beach') provide us a basic linguistic 'map' of the neurological 'map'. And given the way our minds work, we can then use even more abstract and conceptual words ('pleasure', 'comfort') as a higher level linguistic 'map' of the other linguistic 'map', etc.

Given the fact that words function in our consciousness as *a map of reality* (and not even the first level *map*), then words work to provide us a scheme, model, or paradigm *about* that reality. To the extent that the words correspond in an isomorphic way ('form', 'similar') to the territory they represent—they give us an accurate map. To the extent that they do not, they give us a distorted map with significant parts left out (deleted), or with parts over-generalized or messed-up.

Figure 9:1

Evaluative-Based (Meta-linguistics)	Language that describes the meaning, the language, and our feelings, etc., about the experience. Words of the sensory-based words of the... second linguistic map (Meta-words) of the experience.
Sensory-Based (Linguistic Sorting)	Naming and describing words (signifiers); names of objects, entities, categories (nouns); of actions (verbs); qualities (adjectives, 'submodalities') and relationships (prepositions), etc. First linguistic map of the experience.
Neurological (Conscious Experience)	Awareness of experience. What we pay attention to and what we delete. VAK representations of the experience.
Neurological	Processing sense receptors bringing information into our nervous systems (NS).
The Territory	Territory of sensory base reality out there.

NLP began here. Linguist John Grinder had studied, and contributed to the field of transformational grammar for years—a field that sought to understand how the coding, meaning, and significance at the deep structures of experience (at the neurological levels) become transformed into language (at the linguistic levels). Thereafter (1975), he and Bandler put together *the Meta-model of language for therapy.*

They developed this model of language elegance by modeling Fritz Perls and Virginia Satir. Bandler and Grinder noticed their use of certain powerful questions in gathering information and another set of powerful questions that essentially enabled the person to reorganize his internal world. From a linguistic analysis of their language, Bandler and Grinder developed this Meta-model. ('*Meta*' comes from Greek and means 'beyond, over, about, on a different level'.) The Meta-model specifies how we can use language to clarify language. It does so by re-connecting a speaker's language with the experience out of which it came.

> **Bandler and Grinder noticed their use of certain powerful questions in gathering information and another set of powerful questions that essentially enabled the person to reorganize their internal world.**

Obviously, the business of communication involves *language use*—it involves 'sharing the word', and it involves living the word. The more we know about the neuro-linguistic processes at the root of language processing and languaging others and ourselves—the more effective our ability to handle this most incredible tool.

Deep Structure/Surface Structure

The Meta-model provides us with a tool to get to the experience behind a person's words. When we speak, none of us give a complete description of the thoughts behind our words. If we attempted to completely describe our thoughts, we would never finish speaking. Why? Because none of our verbal descriptions can fully or completely (exhaustively) say everything about an experience. As a speaker, we will always have a more complete internal representation of what we wish to communicate than what we can put into words. We inevitably shorten the description.

Now we call the complete internal representation (experience) of what we seek to communicate the 'deep structure'. Most of this deep structure lies in unconscious parts of mind and neurology— some of it at levels *prior* to words, some *beyond* where words can describe. As we seek to present, articulate and clarify our experiences, we do so in what we call 'surface structures'—the words and sentences that represent *transforms* of the deeper levels.

While transformational grammar has not proved adequate to fully explain language acquisition, syntactic structure, etc., the Meta-model does not depend upon the validity or adequacy of transformational grammar. The Meta-model only presupposes that below (or above, depending upon the operational metaphor), there exists another level or layer of abstraction—prior to the surface structure —out of which the surface structure arose.

Because the human nervous system and mind constantly 'leaves characteristics out' (Korzybski) or 'deletes' (Bandler and Grinder) or functions as a 'reducing valve' (Huxley), surface structure as cognitive maps suffers impoverishment. The Meta-model with its challenges involves a process whereby a person expands and extends the cognitive map, making it richer and fuller.

Deletions

Bandler and Grinder noted that in the process of moving from the deep structure in our neurology (our neurological map) to the surface structures that come out of our conscious minds and mouths, we do three things, which they termed 'modeling processes'. For the most part, we do this naturally and apart from consciousness. First, we *delete* much if not most of the material in the deep structure. Every second, approximately two million pieces of information feed into the brain. Obviously, the brain must screen out much information or else we would go crazy. Read the following:

Figure 9:2

> **Paris in the**
> **the spring.**
>
>   **A snake in the**
>   **the grass.**
>
>   **A kick in the**
>   **the rear.**

Lewis and Pucelik (1982) presented this in their treatment of the Meta-model (p. 7). Did you notice as you read that you deleted one of the 'the's in each of those sentences? Unless you put yourself into a detailed state of mind (a proofreader's state of mind) you made sense of the sentence by quickly and unconsciously deleting the second 'the'.

Distortions

Second, we *distort* the meaning and structure of information as we simplify our description of the experience. We alter our perceptions using our brains. A story in Eastern philosophy relates how a man walked along the road and saw a snake. Immediately he yelled, 'Snake!' But then, as he approached it, he saw it more clearly as a rope, and not a snake.

'Beauty' lies in the eye of the beholder. The ability to distort enables us to enjoy works of art, music and literature. Thus we can look at a cloud and turn its vague shapes into animals, people and all kinds of things—we do it by using our brain's power of distortion. Our ability to distort makes it possible for us to have dreams and visions about our desired future.

Generalizations

Third, we *generalize* information. When new learnings come into our brain, our brain *compares* the new information with similar information previously learned. Our minds compare and generalize old similar material with new data. This process allows us to learn quickly. We do not have to relearn old concepts. Our brain utilizes them in new learnings. Although many kinds of cars exist, we relate to them through the category or class that we call 'cars'. Mapping out experiences, events, people, learnings, ideas, etc. through categories enables us to compare, contrast, group, sub-group, etc. This helps us handle increasingly large amounts of information, process information through logical levels, and move into more and more conceptual levels of reality.

While other mapping functions exist, the Meta-model uses these three. They describe the key processes whereby we move from the deep structure within our mind-neurology to our surface structures that show up in our language and languaging. In summary, we delete, distort and generalize information as we create our model of the world.

Meta-model questions *reverse* the process of going from deep structure to surface structure.

What does this Meta-model consist of precisely? It consists of 13 (in this model) language distinctions and 13 sets of questions. These challenging questions inquire about the ill-formedness that shows up in the surface structures and this enables the speaker to restore the material deleted, distorted and generalized. Meta-model questions *reverse* the process of going from deep structure to surface structure. It reverses the abstracting process—we 'de-abstract' via the Meta-model—we take a person *back to experience*.

The Meta-model thus uncovers missing information in the client's communication and model of the world—often crucial information the lack of which causes them to live in the world with an impoverished map. Some ask, 'When do you stop asking Meta-model questions?' Good question. You stop when you have your outcome.

In this work, I will not cover in detail the questions of the Meta-model but will refer the reader to *The User's Manual for the Brain* for a summary of the model. For a more complete understanding of the model and for recent additions to the model I refer the reader to Michael Hall's *The Secrets of Magic*. Herein, we will consider the language distinctions of the Meta-model coupled with the other language distinctions that Bandler and Grinder discovered that Milton Erickson utilized.

Figure 9:3 Chunking Up/Chunking Down

In Trance

General—chunk up—big picture
Questions: What is this an example of?
For what purpose…?
What is your intention?
What does having this give you that is more important?

The Milton Model

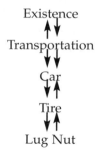

Existence

Transportation

Car

Tire

Lug Nut

The Meta Model

Out Of Trance

Specific—details—chunk down

Questions: What are examples of this?
What specifically?
Any Meta-model question

Why consider the questions of the Meta-model in a book on hypnosis? Good question. After developing the Meta-model, Bandler and Grinder met Milton Erickson, a world-renowned medical hypnotherapist and founder of the American Society for Clinical Hypnosis. Grinder reported that Erickson provided him with the single greatest model he had ever used (O'Connor and Seymour, 1990, p. 119). Erickson opened an entire new area of thought in therapy and communication.

From their study of Erickson, they published *Patterns of the Hypnotic Techniques of Milton H. Erickson Volume I* (1975). Later (1977), with Judith DeLozier, they published *Volume 2*. Bandler and Grinder learned from Erickson the value of trance and altered states in therapy. All of NLP comes from the discoveries of the Meta-model of language and that includes understanding the linguistic structure of Ericksonian hypnosis. Thus, a student of Erickson will greatly benefit from having a basic understanding of the Meta-model.

> **All of NLP comes from the discoveries of the Meta-model of language and that includes understanding the linguistic structure of Ericksonian hypnosis. Thus, a student of Erickson will greatly benefit from having a basic understanding of the Meta-model.**

The Meta-model *steps down to specifics* to recover distorted, generalized and deleted materials; this takes us *out of trance*. The Milton model conversely *chunks up* to make new generalizations, deletions and distortions. Rather than go for specific information, it steps up to general information—to the big picture. The Milton model *mirrors in reverse* the Meta-model (Figure 9:3). So, by actually utilizing the linguistic patterns of the Meta-model in our language and by excluding the questions from the model, we in fact 'send the client' inside to put meaning on the distortions, generalizations and deletions that we are using. After explaining the linguistic structures of the Meta-model patterns, we will give you an example of how these patterns induce trance.

Distortions

1. *Nominalization*

By nominalization we refer to those kinds of nouns that originated from process. They function Meta to experience and symbolize whole chunks of experience. Young (1999) states, 'They are iconic, like the symbols on a computer screen. When you metaphorically 'double-click' on the icon, it opens up to reveal something of the experience(s) it stands for.' Nominalizations take processes and freeze them so that the process movie becomes a still picture. A nominalization can be a word that represents a process, movement, action (verb) or ideas, understandings, and concepts such as memories, rules, principles, values and beliefs.

Linguistically, nominalization refers to changing a deep structure *process* (movement, action, etc.) into a surface structure *static event*. The classic NLP description that tests for a nominalization versus a true noun asks: 'Can you put it in a wheelbarrow?'. If so, you have a noun! If not, then behold—a nominalization! Another way to determine a Nominalization involves seeing if the suspected word will fit in the blank of the following phrase: 'An ongoing_____.' A *process word* like a nominalization will make sense in that syntactic environment whereas a concrete noun will not.

Nominalizations delete large amounts of information. Consider the statement, 'Our poor *relationship* really bothers me'. 'Relationship' functions as a nominalization, even though we generally treat it as a concrete noun. But we cannot see, hear, smell or taste a relationship. We can't put a relationship in a wheelbarrow. Changing the verb 'relating' into the pseudo-noun 'relationship', nominalizes the verb. Other examples of nominalizations: *education, illness, respect, discipline, friendship, decision, love, fear, strategy* and *sensation*.

To challenge nominalizations, we reverse the process. As a person has changed a process into a thing, we now direct him to *change the thing back into a process*. We do that by using the format: 'In what way do you do the process of (nominalization)?'. This question then assists the person to reconnect with the experience in a way that recognizes their role in the process. Examples of nominalizations: 'I have a poor relationship'; 'You have no respect for me'; 'Our system of education...'.

However, in hypnosis, we fill our language with nominalizations for they send the listener 'inside' to put meaning to the words. Indeed, I (BB) illustrate this in class by just speaking nominalizations without giving any context and then I watch the class go into trance as they go inside to put their meanings to words like:

◆　　Education
◆　　Friendship
◆　　Communication
◆　　Love
◆　　Learnings
◆　　Discipline
◆　　Decisions

And, notice, if you paused and put 'your' meaning to each one of those words how you tended to 'go inside' to find that meaning and in going inside you went into a sort of a mild trance, didn't you?

Examples of sentences with nominalizations

I have a poor relationship.
You have no respect for me.
Our system of education stinks.
Communication is a problem in their marriage.
Management made poor decisions.
His desires got him into trouble.
Her behavior is unacceptable.
This exercise will provide you with new insights, and new
　　　understandings.

2. *Mind-Reading*

We engage in mind reading when we think and assert that we know the thoughts, motives, intentions, etc., in another's mind. We do this when we say, 'I know exactly how you feel'. In spite of communicating sympathy, typically such statements trigger pain, resentment, misunderstanding, etc. Mind-reading surface structure reveals much more about *the speaker's internal experience* than the others. Accordingly, when we utter mind-reading statements, we *project* our own perceptions, values, issues, history, etc. Thus, they usually have little to do with the person to whom we speak.

In the Meta-model we would chunk down on mind-reads, 'How specifically do you know how I feel (think, intend, etc.)?'. But in hypnotic languaging we would utilize mind-reads for 'I know you love going into trance, don't you?'.

Examples of Mind-Reads

I know he doesn't care.
She knows better.
I'm sure you're aware. . .
I can tell you don't like me.
He isn't interested.
You think. . . .
You're upset.
I know that you are wondering.

3. *Cause–Effect*

The over-used accusation, 'You *make* me mad!', illustrates a cause–effect statement. This sentence implies that you directly make or cause me to feel mad as if I have no choice in the process. However you create this effect—when you do, I must feel this way. It seems to imply that you have a kind of psychic power over me. Words that indicate the presence of cause–effect statements include: *make, if then, as you... then because*, and almost any present tense verb. I (JB) believe the word 'because' will change more minds than any other word. 'Because . . .?'

To challenge such statements, ask, 'How specifically do I cause you to feel bad?', 'By what process do I "make" you have these feelings, thoughts, or responses?', 'Do you have no choice whatever in how you respond to this stimulus?'. Such responses invite the speaker to expand and enhance his map about cause and effect in human relationships. It empowers the speaker to take responsibility for his own feelings, thoughts and responses. It facilitates the speaker to adopt a more proactive response by exploring his choices.

One of the larger-level purposes of therapy involves empowering a client to recognize their response-able powers and to own their responses as their own. Clients generally feel that they suffer the effects of the causes of others. Effective counseling leads them to realize how they also stand 'at cause'. So we lead them to take control of their own lives and responses as they claim their own powers: the power to think, feel, speak and behave. Examples of cause–effect statements: 'I'm late because of you', 'When you believe in me, I can do it', 'You make me feel _____', 'I would do it, but I'm mad', 'I feel badly that I hurt him'.

Towards the end of this section on Milton model patterns, we will give you some special 'linkage language' to utilize in your languaging. These linguistic structures provide great linguistic tools to utilize in directionalizing your language towards a specific mutually agreed on outcome. Cause–effect and complex equivalence, which we will consider next, provide an excellent tool in linking one thought to another thought in your language. As an example, consider the following statement utilizing nominalizations and mind-reads with a cause–effect linkage:

> You say you and your husband have poor communication [*nominalization*]. Now, I know [*mind–read*] you want to communicate well with your husband. And because [*cause–effect*] you love your husband very much and because [*cause–effect*] you wish to develop a stronger bond with him, that will cause [*cause–effect*] you to desire knowledge [*nominalization*] about communication [*nominalization*] and that means [*complex*

equivalence] you will be open for any and all avenues in developing your communication [*nominalization*] skills, won't you?

This pattern has other Milton model patterns that we have not yet covered. We have identified in parenthesis those patterns covered so far to give you an example of how you can use these patterns in hypnotic languaging. Note how we used the cause–effect 'cause' to link the thoughts of 'developing a stronger bond' with the thought of 'desiring knowledge about communication'. And, we used the complex equivalence 'that means' to link that further with the thought of being open for other 'avenues in developing communication skills'.

Examples of Cause–Effect

I'm late because of you.
When you believe in me, I can do it.
You make me feel _____.
I would do it, but I'm mad.
I feel badly that I hurt him.
Just asking that question *you begin to understand*.
You will begin to relax as you learn the Meta-model.
Since you're reading this sentence, you can think of several more
        examples.
Because _____.

4. Complex Equivalence

We generate a complex equivalence whenever we use a part of an experience (an aspect of the external behavior, EB) to become equivalent to the whole of its meaning (our internal state, IS). Thus when we become aware of the external cue, we assume the meaning of the whole experience. 'You did not tell me that you love me this morning; you just don't love me anymore.' Here a person has equated certain *external behaviors* (saying words that express love to someone) and an *internal state* (feeling loved). The construction of complex equivalences utilizes words of equation: *is, that means, equals*, any *to be* verb, etc. A person makes one external phenomenon identical with another internal phenomenon.

We challenge complex equivalence by asking about the equation, 'How specifically does my not telling you that I love you [*EB*] mean that I don't love you anymore [*IS*]?' 'Have I ever failed to tell you that I loved you and yet you knew that I truly did love you?' Such questioning enables the speaker to identify the complex equivalent belief and recover additional material deleted and distorted. 'When I saw Joe's face turn red [*EB*], I knew he was angry [*IS*].' This complex equivalence (CEq.) leads to mind-reading (M-R). 'When you raised your voice [*EB*], it means you are angry' leads to a cause–effect (C–E).

In complex equivalence we have mentally created a relationship between a word or words and some experience which those words name. Lewis and Pucelik (1982) explain:

> For every word learned, everyone has a somewhat different internal experience. These specific experiences associated with words are called Complex Equivalents. Usually, the subtleties between people's understanding of words are irrelevant. However, there are words that sometimes lead to misunderstanding between people. Words like *love, relationship, partnership, fear, power, trust, respect*, and any expressions linked with a person's perception of himself and the environment are critical to the process of communication... (p. 27)

In their excellent work, *Ericksonian Approaches: A Comprehensive Manual* (1999), Battino and South state, 'The difficulty with Complex Equivalences is that people actually believe the two parts are linked and behave accordingly, but without checking the equivalences.' (pp. 74–75) In hypnosis, this truth gives complex equivalences its power. Note Battino and South's statements:

1.   Complex Equivalences = (is) people actually believe
2.   Two parts = (are) linked and behave accordingly

In the process of defining the problem of the ill formedness of complex equivalences, the authors in fact utilize the 'hypnotic effect' of complex equivalence in describing the ill formedness of the structure. Now, whether or not the authors realized consciously their use of complex equivalence, we don't know. However, as mentioned earlier with cause–effect statement, complex equivalences provide excellent 'linkage language' in linking the listener's experience from one communication to the other as Battino and South have here utilized. And, knowing this, *that means* you can utilize the hypnotic effect of complex equivalence in your languaging, doesn't it?

The basic tenet of the general semantics/Korzybskian distinction points out the confusing of the map and territory. Get someone to confuse the two and he will respond to his map as if it was real. In Meta-states we would say that he outframes one idea with another idea of reality as being undeniable. This confusion will of course govern his response. In utilizing complex equivalence in our hypnotic languaging, the hypnotherapist directs the listener in creating new and, hopefully, more useful maps of their territory. Once installed, the listener will operate off his new map.

Examples of Complex Equivalences

Joe's face is red. That must mean he is angry.
Being here means you will change.
Going to bed early means you will be alert.
You know the answer, so you are competent.
Sitting in this room, you are learning many things.
As you master these skills, you will be a better communicator.
Keeping your eyes open like that means you'll go into trance.
And closing your eyes means you'll go even deeper.
That means…

5. Presuppositions

By the term *presupposition*, we refer to the conceptual and linguistic assumptions that have to exist in order for a statement to make sense. By definition, we do not state our presuppositions—they operate rather as the supporting foundation or context of a given statement. In presuppositions we find the person's beliefs about life, the world, self, others, God, etc. And we all operate from specific presuppositions. So when we learn to listen for presuppositions we can hear a lot about the person's model of the world. presuppositions function similar to mind-reads. They just leave out the 'I know'. Any non-sensory specific language will contain presuppositions.

Presuppositions in language work covertly, indirectly and unconsciously, as we have to accept them and their assumptions in order to make sense of the communication. This fact gives presuppositions their power in hypnotic languaging. In order to make sense out of what we speak, the listener will 'go inside' to gather enough information from his map in order to make the statement make sense. This going inside induces trance and gives an opportunity to the hypnotherapist to implant suggestions.

Presuppositions in language work covertly, indirectly and unconsciously, as we have to accept them and their assumptions in order to make sense of the communication. This fact gives Presuppositions their power in hypnotic languaging.

A presupposition can operate positively as with the fundamental Christian belief that God loves every person. And some presuppositions can impose limitations on us. Many presuppositions that limit us begin with *'why'* questions. We can also learn to listen for such terms as: *since, when, if,* etc.

The sentence: 'Why don't you work harder?' presupposes that the recipient does not work hard enough. 'If you only knew, you would understand my pain' presupposes the recipient does not understand the speaker's pain.

To challenge a presupposition, inquire about the assumptions in the statement. 'What leads you to believe that I don't work hard enough? Hard enough according to what standard?'; 'What leads you to believe that I don't know your pain?', 'How specifically do you assume I need to work harder?', or, 'How would you like me to specifically understand your pain?'. What Presuppositions lie in this? 'You have learned a lot about Presuppositions.' 'How excited do you now feel having learned about the Meta-model and its powerful questions?' 'When do you think you would best like to study and practice learning the Meta-model to become even more proficient?'

In utilizing presupposition hypnotically, consider the first two sentences in the pattern in chapter 6 called, 'Status Quo Foe: Noticing Options For Change':

> 'Some things change or evolve over time. After they become different or modified you may wonder how much sooner it could have been what it is now.'

What do these two statements presuppose?

1.   There exists something called 'things' (which is a big nominalization, by the way). It is a Presupposition of existence.

2.   These things 'change' or 'evolve' over 'time'.

3.   There is something called 'time' which is a major nominalization.

4.   In the process of changing or evolving these 'things' they become 'different' or 'modified'. Note how much information is deleted from these broad generalizations.

5.   There is somebody referred to as 'you', another presupposition of existence.

6.   And, 'you may wonder' which presupposes that you may choose to wonder but you may not as well. 'Wonder' functions as a presupposition of awareness in that it draws attention. This gives the client choice, which we highly recommend in doing hypnosis.

7.   Using the temporal presupposition 'sooner', the pattern suggests that the change could have taken place much sooner than it did 'now' which is another temporal presupposition presupposing that the change had already taken place.

You may find other presuppositions in those two sentences, but hopefully these will give you some idea of their power.

Examples of Presuppositions

We have talked about presuppositions.
You are learning about the Meta-model and the powerful
    questions the Meta-model gives us.
If you would study and practice, you would learn the Meta-model.
You can do this even better.
You are changing all the time.
How else do you *go into trance*?
You're seeing things differently now.
You'll be able to learn even more tomorrow.
You realize you have more resources than ever before.
You can easily move in the direction of your past memories.
Most of the examples of this pattern will be written here by you.
You are learning many things.

Generalizations

6. *Universal Quantifiers*

A universal quantifier refers to the set of words that make a universal generalization. It implies a state of absoluteness—of 'all-ness'. In this generalization we make one category represent a whole group. Thus we move from 'Dad abused me at seven years of age', to 'Men always abuse'. This statement generalizes from a particular to the whole class. Generalizations have no reference point. They are intentionally vague.

Universal quantifiers consist of such words as: *all, never, every, always* and *none*. Such words do not leave room for any exceptions. By definition they express a limited mindset. The Meta-model challenge to a universal quantifier involves simply repeating the word back to the person in the form of a question. To 'All men are abusers' we could respond: 'All?' Another challenge involves asking if the speaker has *ever* met a man who did *not* abuse. This challenge brings out the absurdity of the universal quantifier. Examples are: 'All Christians are hypocrites', 'Every politician is a liar', 'Everyone on welfare is lazy'.

John's pattern 'Next: The "Next" Step in Obtaining Your Desired Outcome' (chapter 5) begins with the phrase, 'You can look in your past to notice *all* the steps, one after another, a series of nexts leading you up to here. . .' and concludes with the statement, 'And now simply allow your mind to inform *all* of you what to do next.' The word *all* functions as a universal quantifier excluding any other possibilities. And, as we say in the Southeastern United States, '"You all", know that Universal Quantifiers includes everything and excludes nothing'. And, this fact makes them quite useful to the hypnotherapist.

Examples of Universal Quantifiers

All Christians are hypocrites.
Every politician is a liar.
Everyone on welfare is lazy.
Nobody's perfect.
Everything is wonderful.
We are all in trance now.
There is always tomorrow.
Everybody knows this part is easy.
One can never know all there is to know.
All of the people doing this process are learning many new things.
And all the things, all the things…

7. *Modal Operators*

This linguistic distinction refers to our *mode* whereby we *operate* in the world. Do we operate from a mental world of *laws* (should, must, have to); do we operate from a world of *opportunities* (possible, possible to, can); do we operate from a world of *obligations* (ought, should); or *empowerment* (dare, want to, desire to), etc? In other words these modal operator terms define the boundaries of our model of the world and our style of operation. This suggests, as do all of the Meta-model distinctions, that we can actually learn to *hear people's belief systems* in their talk! NLP assumes that our language reveals and prescribes the quality and limits of our belief systems.

So words like *can* and *cannot*, *should* and *should not* reveal personal beliefs about what we can or cannot do in life. Now modal operators come in several categories. We have the modal operators of necessity, of possibility, impossibility, empowerment, identity, choice, etc. These modes show up in words like *can/cannot*, *possible/impossible*, *am/am not*, and *will/will not*, etc.

Listening for such words informs us what a client believes stands as possible or impossible in his world. 'I can't change my beliefs', 'I can't learn efficiently', 'I can't imagine saying that'. Such language not only describes his limits, it creates such limitations. Modal operators of *possibility* tell us what a person believes possible.

The Meta-model challenge to this goes: 'What would happen if you did change that belief?'. Or, 'What stops you from doing that?'.

Fritz Perls reframed 'I can't...' by saying, 'Don't say I can't, say I won't'. If a client accepted that statement, he moves from no choice to choice, from effect of a problem to the cause of such. All of therapy has to do with putting the client *at cause*. The presupposition in the phrase, 'Don't say I can't, say I won't', assumes that the client can choose.

Necessity words include: *must/must not*, *should/should not*, *ought/ought not*, *have to*, *need to* and *it is necessary*. These describe a model of the world that believes in necessity. Such words define some governing rule the person operates from. Often these rules limit behavior. Telling children that they *should* do their homework can induce a state of guilt (pseudo-guilt). Modal operators of necessity work wonderfully for creating such guilt. Yet if guiltiness doesn't strike you as a particularly resourceful place to come from for studying, instead of telling children that they *should* do their homework, we can tell them that they *can* do their homework. 'And I *get* to help you with it'.

The Meta-model challenge to a modal operator of necessity: 'What would happen if you did/didn't...?'. 'I *should* go to church!': response: 'What would happen if you did go?'. This will elicit specific reasons why they should go to church. The question goes to the deep structure and facilitates the person to recover effects and outcome. It moves the client into the future. Examples: 'I really should be more flexible at times like this', 'I ought to go back to school', 'I have to take care of her', 'You should learn'.

These questions come from Cartesian logic. One can introduce this unique form of questioning by saying, 'You have been thinking about this one way for quite a while and your thinking hasn't changed. May I suggest another line of thinking? [Get her agreement either verbally on non-verbally.] What would happen if you did change that belief?', etc.

Examples of Modal Operators of Necessity

I really should be more flexible at times like this.
I ought to go back to school.
You should not hurry into trance just yet.
You shouldn't go into trance too quickly, now.
You must be getting this now ... at some level ....
I have to take care of her.
You should learn.

Examples of Modal Operators of Possibility/Impossibility

I can't learn.
I couldn't tell him what I think.
You could learn this now.
You could write this down ... or not.
You could feel more and more peaceful.
You can change overnight.
You may hear the words of wisdom.
It's possible to learn everything easily and quickly.
You could come up with a few more examples, now.
You can learn.

Chaining Modal Operators in Hypnotic Languaging

> **Because modal operators define our model of the world and the boundaries of our belief system, they provide the hypnotherapist with some very useful linguistic structures in directionalizing perception.**

Because modal operators define our model of the world and the boundaries of our belief system, they provide the hypnotherapist with some very useful linguistic structures in directionalizing perception. Due to their usefulness, we are including an extensive list of modal operators. These come from Tad James' Master Practitioner Training Manual. Note the addition of the improbability/probability category to the usual NLP possibility/ necessity categories.

Tad has ingeniously added these modal operators because they tend to operate 'in-between' the modal operator of impossibility and the modal operator of possibility. NLP has a pattern called 'chaining anchors' to move a client from a problem state to a resource state. The uniqueness of this pattern lies in its effectiveness in moving a client to a resource state that lies conceptually quite a distance from a problem state. Theoretically, we use it because making the jump from the problem state to the resource state is such a big jump for the client that one needs to create a chain of intermediate states so as to lead the client through a gradation of states towards and to the outcome state.

An example would be in moving from a stuck state to a motivated state. For many clients who do 'stuck' really well, such a jump would not work in utilizing the traditional collapsing anchor model that moves the client from problem state directly to resource state. However, by creating a chain of intermediate states, one can move the client to the state of motivation. An example may go something like this:

1.   Present state (stuck)
2.   Intermediate state #1 (fear—of remaining stuck)
3.   Intermediate state #2 (calm)
4.   Intermediate state #3 (security)

5. Intermediate State #4 (excitement)
6. Desired state #5 (motivation)

Modal operators provide an excellent tool for the hypnotherapist to 'transition' a client from the problem state to the resource state. The modal operators of probability provide the intermediate states. Suppose a client says, 'I can't get unstuck'. Now in devising a chain of modal operators, listen careful to the client and feed back (pace) his modal operators. Using the above example the hypnotherapist could say,

> Now, I know you believe you can't get unstuck. Just suppose that you *could* get unstuck because you are *fearful* of remaining stuck the remainder of your life. And as you think about it, just *pretend* that you are becoming *calm* about your fear as you know you *deserve* to be *secure* in your own resources *daring* to get *excited* about the possibilities for yourself in becoming more *motivated* about what you *wish* to do for you *ought* to be *motivated* as you *choose* to do those things in your life that you *are able* to do and know you *can* do and in fact you *will be motivated* doing them as you see yourself having your outcome, now.

More Modal Operators with Probability

Negative Necessity	Necessity
Doesn't allow	Allow
Don't have to	Got to
Got to not	Have to
It's not time	It's time
Must not	Must
Not necessary	Necessary
Ought not	Need to
Shouldn't	Ought to
Supposed not to	Should
	Supposed to

Improbability	Probability
Couldn't	Could
Don't dare to	Dare to
Don't deserve	Deserve
Don't let	Had better
Don't prefer	Let
Don't pretend	May
Don't wish	Might
Had better not	Prefer
May not	Pretend
Might not	Wish
Wouldn't	Would

Impossibility	Possibility
Am not	Able to
Can't	Am
Doesn't permit	Can
Don't choose to	Choose to
Don't decide	Decide
Don't intend	Do
Impossible	Intend
Try not	It is possible
Unable to	Permit
Won't	Try
	Will

8. *Lost Performative*

When we *perform* upon our world with value judgments, we speak about important values that we believe in. But in a *lost performative* we have stated a value judgment while deleting the performer (speaker) of the value judgment. As a vague value judgment, a lost performative will push the person into the direction you wish for them to go. 'You don't love me'. Note that the value judgment leaves off the name of the person doing the judging but it directs attention to 'love me'.

'Boys shouldn't cry', 'If you're going to do something, give it your best', 'That is a stupid thing you just did'. In these sentences the speaker has made a value judgment about something. Yet statements fail to inform us *who* said such a thing or where the person got that value judgment.

To challenge a lost performative and restore the deleted and distorted material, ask: 'Who says boys shouldn't cry?', 'Who evaluates my actions as stupid?', 'According to whom do you say such a thing?'. Or even more succinctly, ask, 'Says who?'. These questions require that the speaker access more information in the deep structure and identify the source of the judgments. Until we identify the source, we will lack the ability to challenge the statement's validity. Examples: 'Oh, it's not important anyway', 'It's not good to be strict', 'And, it is a good thing to wonder'.

How do we utilize lost performatives hypnotically? Politicians as a rule utilize hypnotic languaging patterns quite extensively. Lost performatives seem to be one of their favorites. How many times do you hear something like this, 'The American people do not want to cut taxes at the cost of Social Security going bankrupt'? Note first that the term 'American people' functions as a universal quantifier. The sentence as a whole is a value judgment but the person(s) doing the judging is left out—lost performative. The term 'American people' is a broad generalization that deletes every American that disagrees with that statement. Everyone understands that, don't they?

Examples of Lost Performatives

Oh, it's not important anyway.
It's not good to be strict.
That's too bad.
Today is a great day.
No one should judge others.
That's perfect!
It's really good that you say that.
One doesn't have to ....
And, it is a good thing to wonder.

Deletions

9. *Simple Deletions*

A simple deletion occurs when the communicator leaves out information about a person, thing or relationship.

Examples of Simple Deletions

I am uncomfortable.
I feel afraid.
I am hurting.
I feel alone.
I don't know.

Hypnotically, by utilizing simple deletions, the hypnotherapist forces the listener into 'filling in' the deleted material. Again, this forces the listener to do a transderivational search for meaning to the deleted material which induces trance.

10. *Comparative Deletions*

In a comparative deletion someone makes a comparison, but deletes the specific persons, things, or items compared or the standard by which the speaker makes the comparison. Words like *better, best, further, nearer, richer, poorer, more, less, most, least, worse,* etc, provide cues of comparative deletions. What you compare to functions as a presupposition and the other person's unconscious mind will fill in what's missing.

'He is much better off'. The challenge: 'Better off than who?', 'Better off according to what standard?'. Other examples of statements with comparative deletions: 'She's a better person', 'He is the best student in the class', 'She is the least likely person I know to have succeeded', 'It is more or less the right thing to do'.

Examples of Comparative Deletions

He is the best student in the class.
She is the least likely person I know to have succeeded.
And it is more or less the right thing to do.

11. *Lack of Referential Index or Unspecified Nouns and Verbs*

By *referential index* we refer to the person or thing that does or receives the action from the verb in the statement. When a sentence lacks a referential index, it fails to specify by name, term or phrase what it references—whom it speaks about. It fails to specify or point to a specific person or group. The pronouns (one, it, they, people, etc.) are unspecified. Crucial material from the deep structure that completes the meaning has been deleted.

Listen for words like *one, they, nobody* and *this*: 'They did not come to the meeting'. Here the speaker failed to specify the subject of the verb. To challenge and recover the deleted material, we ask, 'Who, specifically, did not come to the meeting?'.

In the statement, 'Those people hurt me' the noun phrase ('those people') like the unspecified verb ('hurt') lacks a referential index. So we inquire, 'Who specifically hurt you?'. Other examples of this linguistic distinction: 'They don't listen to me', 'Nobody cares anymore', 'This is unheard of', 'One can, you know'.

Examples of Lack of Referential Indices

They don't listen to me.
Nobody cares anymore.
This is unheard of.
One can, you know.

In hypnotic languaging, by deleting the referential index, the listener will 'go inside' and associate either himself or someone else in filling in the deletion. This phenomenon gives opportunity to the hypnotherapist to embed suggestions as to 'whom' the lack of Referential Index applies.

12. *Unspecified Verbs*

Unspecified verbs describe vague, non-specific action. Words like *hurt, upset, injure, show, demonstrate, care* and *concern* certainly describe action, a process, a set of events or experiences—but they have left out so much of the specific information about the action that we cannot make a clear representation in our mind about that action. She says, 'He hurt me', but we don't know if he slapped her, left her waiting at the mall, molested her, insulted the pie she baked, etc.

We recover such deleted material by asking, 'How did he hurt you exactly?', 'Who specifically hurt you?'. If we fail to ask for the deleted information, we run the risk of inventing it in our own minds! While we may make good guesses if we know enough of the context and background, we may also make guesses that miss the other person's meaning by light years.

When we hear a sentence with an unspecified verb ('She misunderstood me'), the potential exists for much misunderstanding, because we can interpret it in many different ways. The questions will connect the person more fully to his experience. In terms of well-formedness we do not provide a sufficient enough linguistic 'map' for the other person to get a clear message. Examples are: 'You don't care about me', 'I am upset', 'He doesn't show me any concern'.

Examples of Unspecified Verbs

You don't care about me.
I upset my mother.
He doesn't show me any concern.
I was wondering.
If only you knew.
You may discover.
And you can learn this.

When the hypnotherapist does not specify the verb, this forces the listener to do a mind read and to specify the verb from his own trandsderivational search thus inducing trance.

The Milton Model: *Specific Language Patterns for Artful Vagueness*

As we have said before, the Meta-model *steps down to specifics* to recover distorted, generalized and deleted materials; this takes us *out of trance*. The Milton model conversely *chunks up* to make new generalizations, deletions and distortions. Rather than go for specific information, it steps up to general information—to the big picture. The Milton model *mirrors in reverse* the Meta-model (Figure 9:3).

> **Expect to find lots of distortions, generalizations, and deletions in this model. Here we intentionally use language to give the client room to fill in the pieces.**

Expect to find lots of distortions, generalizations, and deletions in this model. Here we intentionally use language to give the client room to fill in the pieces. We provide an open frame with little context so that the client's unconscious mind will activate an internal search. General language inherently induces one to go into a trance on this search. So the language patterns within the Milton model facilitate this process.

> **Because the Milton model mirrors in reverse the Meta-model, we put a person in trance *by using the Meta-model violations*.**

Because the Milton model mirrors in reverse the Meta-model, we put a person in trance *by using the Meta-Model violations*. Here we do not ask questions—questions invite the mind to come up (into up-time). The following illustrates using Meta-Model violations creatively to induce a trance state:

> I know (mind read) that you have come to gain new learnings (nominalization) about a great many subjects (unspecified noun) of significance to you. And, it is a good thing to learn (lost performative), to really learn.... For, as you gain new learnings (presupposition), you have already begun to change (cause–effect) and I don't know how you *feel that*,

now... but you can. And, the fact that you have begun to change in ever so slight ways means that healing (complex equivalence) has begun. And you might experience these changes (presuppositions) by how you feel or just by how you talk to yourself. Since you have begun to make changes (nominalization), that means all (universal quantifier) other areas needing healing can begin to change (entire sentence— a complex equivalence.). And you can change (modal operator of possibility and unspecified verb), as you should (modal operator of necessity). It is more or less the right thing to do, that is to change (comparative deletion).

In addition to these Meta-model categories, the Milton model offers other categories as detailed below:

1. *Tag Questions*

You can displace resistance from a statement by placing a question after the statement, can't you? The question added at the end draws the conscious mind's attention thereby allowing the other information in the sentence to go directly into the unconscious mind. 'It is OK for me to do that, isn't it?' Tag questions 'tamp down' the suggestion contained at the front part of the sentence into the unconscious mind.

Examples of Tag Questions

Isn't it?
Have you?
You know?
Won't you?
Can't you?
Aren't you/we?
That's right?
Don't you know?
Didn't I?
Couldn't you?
Will you?
And you can, can you not?

2. *Pacing Current Experience*

A powerful means of building rapport and inducing trance involves pacing the client's current experience by simply making statements that 'agree with and have similarity with' his ongoing experience. Pacing current experience associates the person into an internal focus.

> You can feel yourself sitting in your chair or lying down ... And, as you read this material, you continue to breathe in and out at first quickly and then as you *take a deep breath* you can become more relaxed, wont you now? The sounds in the room and those that you may hear outside, and the words on the page means that you can go deeper and still deeper into trance.

Of course, noticing the sounds in the room have nothing to do with relaxation *unless* you link the two. So as we talked to your unconscious mind, it could say,

> Yes, now that you mention it, I do hear sounds and I can take a deep breath and of course, this makes the next statement about going into a trance much more believable.

Examples of Pacing Current Experience

You hear my voice.
We are in this group.
You will enjoy it more.
As you notice each blink of your eyes.
As you sit here now you can hear external sounds ...
And you can hear internal sounds...
You can experience being bathed by the light...
As you continue breathing in and out...
You can experience yourself going deeper and deeper into trance.

3. *Double Binds*

'And you can go into a trance now or ten minutes from now and I don't know which you'll do ...'. If your unconscious mind accepted the presupposition of that sentence, you will either have already entered a trance or you will shortly. Double binds have an unspoken presupposition contained within the sentence. Parents seem to have a natural talent at communicating double binds: 'John, when will you do your homework? Before this TV program comes on or as soon as it ends?'. 'Now that you have entered a trance, which arm do you wish to lift?', 'Do you wish your right arm to raise or your left?'. Asking which hand the image will come out on (in the visual squash) illustrates an example of a double bind.

Figure 9:4 Double Binds

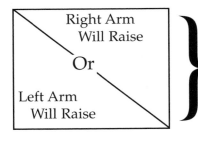

```
Right Arm
Will Raise

Or

Left Arm
Will Raise
```
'Do you wish for your right arm to raise or your left' gives choice as to which arm will raise, but the question presupposes that *one* arm will raise.

Examples of Double Binds

Do you want to begin now, or later?
As you dream, or upon awakening ....
Either before, or after, leaving this room ....
When you go to bed you will either dream, or not.
Will you begin to change now or after this session?

Would you like to quit smoking today or tomorrow?
Would you like to buy the car now, or test drive it first?
You either will or you won't (followed by an unspecified verb).
Take all the time you need to finish up in the next five minutes.
You can change as quickly or as slowly as you want to now.
If you don't write at least one more double bind in the space below
      now, you will either think of one automatically very soon,
      or else wonder when the next one will come to mind, so
      you can write it down then.

4. *Conversational Postulate*

A conversational postulate takes the form of a 'modal operator' question which is actually a command to do something. The answer requires a yes or no response. However, that question seems to bypass the conscious mind and create within the unconsciousness a desire to *do something* about the statement. A classic example is: 'Can you close the door?'. Instead of responding with a 'yes' or 'no', most of us respond by simply closing the door. Such questions avoid authoritarianism.

Examples of Conversational Postulate

Can you imagine this?
Will you just let go now?
Can you picture doing this?
Can you see what I am saying?
Can you reach that level now?
Would it be all right to feel this good?
Do you know that you know it already?
Could you open your mind for a moment?
How easily do you think you can do this?
Can you remember to be kind to yourself?
Does this sound like it will work for you?
Do you feel prepared to sign the contract now?
Do you think you can make the changes you want?

Would you like… to just sit here… and relax now?

Wouldn't you like to just drift into that peaceful state?

Would you mind writing down a couple more conversational postulates here?

5. *Extended Quotes*

Susan said that she heard Dave say that Tad James said, 'I heard Richard say that NLP offers some of the most powerful if not the most powerful tools for personal change available today. And, these tools locate themselves within your unconscious mind. In fact, you have access to them at the unconscious level. Once your conscious mind and unconscious mind gain rapport with each other, then you will have now total access to those resources. That is what Tad said he heard Dave say from what he heard Susan say.'

Many speakers make extensive use of quotes. The use of quotations takes the attention away from the speaker and serves to displace the conscious mind so the information can go into the unconscious mind. The listener accesses a trance by focusing on the quotation as it facilitates an inward focus. Extended Quotes play off our need to make sense out of statements.

Examples of Extended Quotes

Last year, in San Diego, John Grinder was telling us about this African drummer who asked Judy if she had heard the village chief say how easy it is to generate extended quotes.

Last year, I met a woman who said she knew a man who had mentioned that his father told him …

Bob said that in a training four years ago, he had told the story about when Richard Bandler was quoting Virginia Satir, who used to say that …

I was speaking with a friend the other day, who told me of a
conversation she had had with a therapist who told her
about a session he'd had with a client who said …

When I went to Charlotte, North Carolina the other day with
Sam and Doris, one of them told a story about when his
mother would sit down and explain to the children how
father had said …

The other day, a participant in the training told me that her husband said Bob had told him to ask you to write a couple
of extended quotes down right here.

6. *Selectional Restriction Violation*

A selectional restriction violation describes an ill-formed sentence
which ascribes feelings to an animal or some inanimate object:
'Have you ever thought about your pen, typewriter or word pro-
cessor? Just think how many notes it has taken over the years.
How many, I wonder? It knows more than even you know'. 'What
about giving your chair some thought? Don't you know it gets
tired? After all, it has carried your weight for a long time, hasn't
it?'. Such language creates ambiguity in the listener which in turns
creates trance.

Examples of Selectional Restriction Violation

My rock said…
The walls have ears.
That nail hurt my tire.
Flowers like to be picked.
My car knows how to get here.
Put the noise down in your toe.
What did your actions say to you?
Could you open your mind for a moment and just listen to what
the butterfly has to tell you? because the words have
power of their own.

The cat doesn't care about the furniture's outrage from the
       scratching.
As he picked up the spoon, the Jell-O trembled with fear.
And if your pen told us all the things it has learned.
My car loves to go fast when the road beckons.
Do trees cry when they drop their leaves?
Sometime the cookies just call to you.
Do you know what the pen thought?
These walls can tell such stories.
Your pen knows how to write selectional restriction violations
       very easily, if you will just lead it to the lines below now.

In Bandler's Weight Loss Transcript he utilizes the following *selectional restriction violations*:

> 'The furnace inside you …': this refers to the metabolism of the body.

> 'I want to talk to that part of you … or your unconscious.'

> 'And this is what he installs in people ….'

> 'And your brain goes brrrrrrr …'

> 'The box of Godiva chocolates calls out to you.'

7. *Phonological Ambiguities*

Many words have different meanings but sound the same: 'Your nose/knows the truth of this', 'You can be hear/here anytime you wish'. Such language distracts the conscious mind. The client will go into trance while trying to sort out the ambiguities.

Examples of Phonological Ambiguities

you're/your
there/their

here/hear
son/sun
bare/bear bottoms
there's no 'their' in there
He reddened as he read in it.
You are the one who has won.
After all you have learned from the tapes.
And here today as you hear your unconscious mind ....
You can trust *you're unconscious* mind *now*.

8. *Syntactic Ambiguity*

Syntactic ambiguity exists when we cannot immediately determine from the immediate context the function (syntax) of a word.
For instance, 'Hurting people can feel difficult'. Does that sentence
mean that when you meet hurting people they can make this difficult for us emotionally, or does it mean that engaging in the
behavior of hurting people feels like a difficult problem? We can
construct syntactic ambiguities by using *a verb* plus *-ing*. Then you
construct a sentence so that it lacks clarity about whether the *-ing*
word functions as an adjective or as a verb. This phraseology
induces trance in the listener. The listener will go inside trying to
figure out the functions of the language which will deepen the
trance.

Examples of Syntactic Ambiguities

running water
shooting stars
babbling brook
hypnotizing hypnotists can be tricky.

9. *Scope Ambiguity*

Scope ambiguity exists when you cannot determine by context
how much one portion of a sentence applies to another portion:
'The organization consists of healthy men and women'. Do we

mean to imply that just the men have the quality of 'health' or do we mean to include the women as healthy as well? You can construct scope ambiguity by adding an *-ing* on a verb and put an 'and' between the objects. The listener, in attempting to determine what part of the sentence belongs to or modifies what other part of the sentence, will go into trance.

Examples of Scope Ambiguities

Your deep breathing and trance …
Hearing Bob and John …
Yesterday I was driving my car with tennis shoes on.
I was riding my horse with blue jeans on.

10. *Punctuation Ambiguity*

There exist three kinds of punctuation ambiguities. The first involve *run-on sentences*: 'I want you to notice your hand me the book', 'On your arm I see a watch yourself go into trance'. The second form involves *improper pauses*. This form of sentence involves times when you begin a …. uh… sentence and you never quite … uh … finish the … sentence. This causes a forced mind reading and becomes highly trance inducing. Newscaster, Paul Harvey, does this in a marvelous way when he says, '… good … day.' The third type of punctuation ambiguity involves an *incomplete sentence*. In this form you begin a sentence and you never quite… You then go on to another sentence with a totally different thought.

Examples of Run-on Sentences

Let me take your hand me the pen.
See the butterfly drifting over the hilltop is a beautiful valley.
She has freckles on her butt I like her anyway.

Examples of Improper Pauses

My wife left me ... to go to Texas.
I was looking for my tie ... into this thought.
If you hear any ambiguities ... it's all right to write them right here.

Examples of Incomplete Sentences

I just taught .... How is your day going?
He hurt ... She is doing much better.
Let it ... And you will feel much better.

11. *Utilization*

Erickson utilized utilization to its fullest potential. He used every thing the client said. He used every sound and incident in the room. In one of my (BB) trainings a wall chart fell off the wall. Tad James said, 'And old concepts are falling away'. Once when I used hypnosis with a client, I had a relaxation tape playing. Suddenly the tape finished. I knew that in a short moment that the tape player would make a click as it cut off. So, I said, 'In just a moment you will hear a click. And, when you do, that means you will let go of the pain totally and completely'. In a brief moment the player clicked and the client's body jumped as the emotion totally released.

Examples of Utilization

Client: 'I don't think I know'.
Practitioner: 'That's right, you don't think *you know*'.

Client: 'I can't be hypnotized'.
Practitioner: 'That's right. You can't be *hypnotized yet*'.

Client: 'I'm not sold'.
Salesman: 'That's right, because you haven't asked the one
        question yet that will let you be sold'.

12. *Embedded Commands*

Erickson worked as a master at giving the unconscious mind directions through embedded commands. He would *mark out such words* that he wanted to go into the unconscious mind. To give such commands and mark out words, we have to both lower our tone and raise the volume of the voice: '*It is possible for you* to instruct a client's unconscious mind through embedded commands *to get well, now*'.

13. *Analogue Marking*

Erickson would *mark out* the words that he wanted to go into the unconscious mind. *Marking out* refers to emphasizing specific words or phrases. You can mark out certain words by using the same technique of delivering embedded commands by lowering the tone of your voice and by raising the volume of your voice. You can also mark out certain words by moving some part of your anatomy on certain words. For instance, you could raise an eyebrow on certain words thus signaling the listener's unconscious mind that this word is important. Allow your creative mind to give you other ways to *mark out* certain words.

14. *Spell Out Words*

I (JB) believe that by spelling out key words we draw attention to the word we are spelling out. This induces trance. And, you k-n-o-w that spelling out words does induce trance, doesn't it?

15. *Linkage Language*

This refers to the verbal process of describing (pacing) observable and verifiable behavior in the listener. Then, by using a 'linking word', the speaker goes on to describe (leading) the desired behavior. Different people, of course, respond differently to each pattern. Linkage language involves the process of utilization connected to specific linking words.

a. *Conjunctions*

Use a conjunction such as 'and' to link observable behavior and desired experience. The conjunction links the pacing statement to the leading statement ('X' and 'Y'). For example, 'As you sit there, breathing and reading this document and you can begin to breathe more deeply and become more relaxed.' The purpose here involves linking the pacing statement to the leading statement so that the latter seems to follow logically from the former. Thus, the linkage collapses information boundaries to enhance the sense of continuity. Additional pacing statements further enhance the effect ('X' and 'X' and 'X' and 'Y'). Examples are: 'As you sit in your chair (pacing) and read this paper (pacing) and I communicate to you (pacing) and you can breathe deeply and relax more thoroughly (leading).'

b. *Disjunction*

Using the contrasting or negative form of conjunctions can also sometimes achieve the same results ('X' and 'X' and 'X' but 'Y'). Examples are: 'I don't know whether you prefer to continue gazing at this paper (pacing), or whether you'd like to look elsewhere (pacing), or whether you'd like to breathe deeper (pacing), but I do know that your conscious can develop a trance that will fit nicely your present needs (leading).

c. *Adverbial Clauses or Implied Causatives*

Causatives often exist as 'time' words that imply that one event inevitably functions as linked in time with, or caused by the other. Key implied causatives include: (1) *since 'X' then 'Y'*, *since* you are now breathing deeper, you can begin to relax even more; (2) *when 'X' then 'Y'*, *when* you settle comfortably into that chair, you can allow your eyes to slowly close; (3) *while 'X' then 'Y'*, *while* you remember that very special time and place, you can comfortably begin to develop that trance; (4) *after 'X' then 'Y'*, *after* you have become very comfortable, you can begin to allow your trance to develop; and (5) other implied causative words include: *often, as, before, during, following* and *throughout*.

To familiarize yourself with these language patterns, write down five sentences for each. Include the Meta-model violations as well in your exercise. You will find these skills most helpful in all areas of communication and highly useful in public speaking.

Conclusion

'Hypnosis' and trance describes nothing new, odd, occult, strange or mysterious. Our consciousness can 'come up' (up-time) and 'go down' (downtime). And when it goes down inside, we enter into another world, the inner world of meaning, belief, concepts—a world of spirit where we create our neuro-semantic reality.

Nor can we escape from this. We can only effectively develop awareness and understanding of this and how it plays out in communication in everyday life so that we can have more choice and control over it. When we do that, then we can choose our hypnotists well. Then we can know when to 'go into trance' and when to come out! Then we will not allow ourselves to unknowingly or unconsciously receive the onslaught of the bad suggestions that some people forever put out. Then we can know how to dehypnotize ourselves from the dysfunctional negative suggestions leftover (in our heads) from childhood. Then we can take a proactive stance in communicating positive and enhancing suggestions for ourselves and others. This empowers us in communicating professionally and consciously.

Figure 9.5: Summary of Milton Model Language

Milton Model Language Patterns Using Meta-Model Violations

1. Nominalization
2. Mind-Reading
3. Cause–Effect
4. Complex Equivalence
5. Presuppositions
6. Universal Quantifiers
7. Modal Operators of Necessity/Possibility
8. Lost Performative
9. Simple Deletions
10. Comparative Deletions
11. Lack of Referential Index
12. Unspecified Verbs

Milton Model Continued

1. Tag Questions
2. Pacing Current Experience
3. Double Binds
4. Conversational Postulate
5. Extended Quotes
6. Selectional Restriction Violation
7. Phonological Ambiguities
8. Syntactic Ambiguity
9. Scope Ambiguity
10. Punctuation Ambiguity
11. Utilization
12. Embedded Commands
13. Analogue Marking
14. Spell Out Words

Linkage Languaged

15.a   Conjunctions 'X' and 'Y'
15.b   Disjunctions 'X' and 'X' and 'X' but 'Y'
15.c   Adverbial Clauses (implied causatives)
15.c   (1) Since 'X' then 'Y'
15.c   (2) When 'X' then 'Y'
15.c   (3) While 'X' then 'Y'
15.c   (4) After 'X' then 'Y

Bibliography

Bandler, Richard and Grinder, John (1975) *The Structure of Magic, Volume 1: A Book about Language and Therapy*. Palo Alto, CA: Science and Behavior Books.

Bandler, Richard and Grinder, John (1975) *Patterns of the Hypnotic Techniques of Milton H. Erickson, M.D., Volume 1*. Cupertino, CA: Meta Publications.

Bandler, Richard, Delozier, Judith and Grinder, John (1977) *Patterns of the Hypnotic Techniques of Milton H. Erickson, M.D., Volume 2*. Cupertino, CA: Meta Publications.

Bateson, Gregory (1972) *Steps to an Ecology of Mind*. New York: Ballantine.

Battino, Rubin and South, Thomas L. (1999) *Ericksonian Approaches: A Comprehensive Manual*. Carmarthen: Crown House Publishing Limited.

Bodenhamer, Bob (1995) 'Taking a Bitter Root to Jesus', *Anchor Point* (April): 20-4.

Bodenhamer, Bob (1995) 'The Meta-YES, and Meta-NO Pattern', *Anchor Point* (April): 20-5.

Bodenhamer, Bob and Hall, Michael (1999) *The User's Manual for the Brain*. Carmarthen: Crown House Publishing Limited.

Bodenhamer, Bob and Hall, Michael (1997) *Time-Lining: Patterns for Adventuring in 'Time'*. Carmarthen: Crown House Publishing Limited.

Burton, John (1998) 'I Never Met a Meta-State Without a Program', *Anchor Point* (October): 26–9.

Burton, John (n.d.) 'States of Equilibrium'; unpublished manuscript.

Chong, Dennis and Chong, Jennifer (1991) *Don't Ask Why: A Book About the Structure of Blame, Mad Communication and Miscommunication*. Oakville, ON: C-Jade Publishing.

Festinger, Leon (1957) *A Theory of Cognitive Dissonance*. Stanford, CA: Stanford University Press.

Gilligan, Stephen (1987) *Therapeutic Trances: The Cooperative Principle in Ericksonian Hypnotherapy*. Levittown, NY: Brunner-Mazel.

Hall, L. Michael (1995) *Meta-states: A Domain of Logical Levels, Self-reflexive Consciousness in Human States of Consciousness*. Grand Junction, CO: ET Publications.

Hall, L. Michael (1996) *The Spirit of NLP: The Process, Meaning and Criteria for Mastering NLP*. Carmarthen: Crown House Publishing Ltd.

Hall, L. Michael (1997) 'Recognizing the Meta-levels of Beliefs, Part 1', *Anchor Point* (November): 13–19.

Hall, L. Michael (1998) *The Secrets of Magic: Communicational Excellence For the 21st Century*. Carmarthen: Crown House Publishing.

Hall, L. Michael and Bodenhamer, Bob (1997a) *Figuring Out People: Design Engineering with Meta-programs*. Carmarthen: Crown House Publishing.

Hall, L. Michael and Bodenhamer, Bob (1997b) *Mind Lines: Lines for Changing Minds*. Grand Junction, CO: ET Publications.

Hall, L. Michael and Bodenhamer, Bob. (1999). Structure of Excellence: Unmasking the Meta-levels of 'Submodalities'. Grand Junction, CO.: ET Publications.

Hearst, E. (1977) 'Fundamentals of Learning and Conditioning', in R. C. Atkinson, R. J. Hernstein, G. Lindzey and R. D. Luce (eds) *Stevens' Handbook of Experimental Psychology*. New York: Wiley.

Korzybski, Alfred (1933/1994) *Science and Sanity: An Introduction to Non-Aristotelian Systems and General Semantics,* (4th and 5th edn) Lakevill, CN: International Non-Aristotelian Library Publishing Co.

Lewis, Bryon A. and Pucelik, Frank (1982) *Magic Demystified: A Pragmatic Guide to Communication and Change.* Portland, Oregon: Metamorphous Press.

Loevinger, Jane (1976) *Ego Development: Conceptions and Theories.* San Francisco, CA: Jossey-Bass.

O'Connor, Joseph and Seymour, John (1990) *Introducing Neuro-Linguistic Programming: Psychological Skills for Understanding and Influencing People.* London: Thorsons.

Piaget, Jean (1965) *The Child's Conception of the World.* New Jersey: Littlefield, Adams & Company.

Rossi, Ernest, Ryan, Margaret O. and Sharp, Florence A. (1983) *Healing in Hypnosis: The Seminars, Workshops, and Lectures of Milton H. Erickson, Volume 1.* New York: Irvington Publishers.

Watzlawick, Paul, Weakland, John and Fisch, Richard (1974) *Change Principles of Problem Formation and Problem Resolution.* New York: W.W. Norton & Co.

Wertheimer, Max (1912) 'Experimentelle Studien Uber das Sehen von Bewegung', *Zeitschrift fur Psychologie* 60: 312–78.

Index